A Patient's Guide to Mesothelioma

By Joseph W. Belluck

Belluck & Fox, LLP

A Patient's Guide to Mesothelioma

Joseph W. Belluck

Belluck & Fox, LLP
546 Fifth Ave, 4th Floor
New York, NY 10036
Toll-free: 877-637-6843

Visit our websites:

www.belluckfox.com
www.mesotheliomahelp.net

© Joseph W. Belluck, 2018
All rights reserved. No part of this publication may be reproduced, in whole or in part, without the express written consent of the publisher.

Belluck, Joseph W.
A Patient's Guide to Mesothelioma

ISBN 9781484141366
Health & Fitness / Diseases / Cancer

Table of Contents

Introduction: How to Use This Book   1

Chapter 1: Understanding What Mesothelioma Is   3
- Who's at Risk   3
- How Your Respiratory System Works   5
- Types of Mesothelioma   7
- Mesothelioma Stages and Cell Types   8
- Other Asbestos-Related Lung Diseases   10

Chapter 2: What Is Asbestos?   12
- Types of Asbestos and Their Uses   12
- Discovery of the Health Hazards of Asbestos   14

Chapter 3: Diagnosing Mesothelioma   19
- Mesothelioma Symptoms   19
- Diagnosing Mesothelioma   22
- Imaging Tests   23
- Taking Biopsies   29

Chapter 4: Treating Mesothelioma   34
- Surgery   35
- Chemotherapy   39
- Radiation Therapy   45
- New Therapies   46
- Clinical Trials   47
- Finding a Doctor and Treatment Center   48

Chapter 5: Living With Mesothelioma   50
- Taking Care of Your Physical Health   50
- Dealing with the Emotional Impact   55
- Considering Hospice Care   59

Chapter 6: Exploring Your Legal Rights and Options	61
    Filing a Timely Claim	61
    Choosing an Attorney	62
    Checking Out Financial Assistance Options	65

Chapter 7: How the Claims Process Works	73
    Stages of a Lawsuit	73

Chapter 8: Other Legal Considerations	80
    Advance Health Care Directives	80
    Wills	82
    Other Important Papers	83

Glossary	84

Appendix A: Mesothelioma Specialists	93

Appendix B: Personal Medical Journal	112

Appendix C: Mesothelioma Treatment Record	132

Appendix D: Records	141

About Belluck & Fox	145

Introduction

How to Use This Book

Families can have a tough time coping with mesothelioma and other asbestos-related illnesses. Because these diseases are relatively rare, you may feel isolated. And your legal options can be complex and confusing.

We have produced this handbook to help answer your questions about the medical and legal aspects of mesothelioma and asbestos-related diseases. The medical and legal aspects of mesothelioma are connected because mesothelioma is an entirely preventable environmental illness caused only by exposure to asbestos.

Written in plain English, with easy-to-understand definitions of technical terms right in the text, this book is designed to serve two purposes: It's a reference for you to turn to with your medical and legal questions, as well as a personal journal for you to track your treatments and other important information in one convenient place.

The book is divided into three sections. Chapters 1 through 5 cover the medical side of mesothelioma and asbestos-related disease. Chapters 6 through 8 help you navigate and understand your legal options if you (or a loved one) suffer from the effects of asbestos exposure. In the back of the book, you'll find a glossary, a list of doctors and treatment centers that specialize in mesothelioma and related diseases, and useful charts and checklists for keeping track of your symptoms, treatments, and important documents and records.

You don't have to read this book cover-to-cover, or even in order. Each chapter is written so that you can turn directly to the information that's most important to you.

Cross-references to other chapters are provided so you can easily find answers to your questions. And each chapter includes a page or two for you to make your own notes.

Mesothelioma is a relatively rare but serious illness, and it's natural to feel overwhelmed when it strikes close to home. But you don't have to face this life-changing diagnosis – or its consequences – alone. Use this book to get the information you need to make informed choices about your medical care and legal rights. And visit us online at www.mesotheliomahelp.net for additional assistance.

Chapter 1

Understanding What Mesothelioma Is

Mesothelioma is a rare form of cancer that arises in the *mesothelium*, a thin membrane that protects your internal organs and allows them to move freely without damage-causing friction. You have several of these membranes in your body: the *pleura* surround the lungs; the *peritoneum* protects your abdominal cavity (stomach, intestines, and other organs); and the *pericardium* envelops your heart.

Mesothelioma can occur in any of these membranes, but pleural mesothelioma is by far the most common, accounting for about 70 percent of all mesothelioma cases. Although some people may have a genetic predisposition for developing mesothelioma, nearly all cases arise from exposure to asbestos. Men typically are at greater risk than women, but women also get this disease.

This chapter provides an overview of mesothelioma, starting with a look at who's at risk for developing mesothelioma, how your respiratory system works and how mesothelioma affects your body. Look for cross-references to other chapters for more detailed information.

Who's at Risk

Between 2,500 and 3,000 new cases of mesothelioma are diagnosed each year. Anyone who has been exposed to asbestos is at risk for developing mesothelioma, and, although your risk increases with the length of time you were exposed to asbestos, even small exposures to asbestos can cause mesothelioma.

Ironically, your risk also increases with the length of time that elapses after your exposure to asbestos. Mesothelioma has a very long *latency period* – that is, the period between exposure to asbestos and the onset of symptoms of the disease.

Mesothelioma typically doesn't appear until at least a decade after asbestos exposure; in some cases, the latency period has been 50 years or longer.

Sometimes, mesothelioma results from exposure to naturally occurring asbestos, but the most common causes are exposure to asbestos in the workplace or from products used in the home (see Chapter 2 for examples of such products). Spouses and family members of workers also may have been exposed to asbestos dust and fibers from the clothing the workers wore home from the job site.

Here are some quick facts about mesothelioma and risk factors:

- Men are more commonly diagnosed than women, because men more typically worked in jobs where they were exposed to asbestos. These high-risk jobs include electricians, shipyard workers, factory workers, pipefitters, oil refinery workers, auto mechanics, machinists, and steel workers. (See Chapter 2 for more on how asbestos was used and the most dangerous jobs relating to asbestos exposure.) Older men account for more than 90 percent of all new mesothelioma diagnoses each year. Although no one knows exactly why, Caucasian men are statistically more likely to develop the disease than African-American or Hispanic men.

- Women who worked in factories had increased direct exposure to asbestos and are more likely to be diagnosed with mesothelioma later in life.

- Women whose husbands, fathers, or other household members worked in high-exposure jobs also are at risk of developing mesothelioma from secondary exposure to the asbestos dust and fibers on work clothes. Children in these homes also are at risk from secondary exposure.

- People who used asbestos-containing products in their homes are at increased risk of developing mesothelioma.

- Because of mesothelioma's long latency period, people over the age of 50 are more likely to be diagnosed with the disease. Most mesothelioma diagnoses come in patients between the ages of 50 and 70; those who are diagnosed earlier may have a better chance of long-term survival.

- People serving as first responders – fire-fighters, police officers, rescue workers and recovery personnel – may be exposed to asbestos at disaster sites, such as the World Trade Center.
- Armed service personnel, especially those serving on ships in the Navy or Coast Guard, also are at higher risk of developing mesothelioma.

How Your Respiratory System Works

Your respiratory system takes in oxygen and releases carbon dioxide, while filtering the air you take in to remove irritants and to control temperature and moisture levels. To accomplish all this, your respiratory system consists of several parts (see Figure 1-1):

- The *epiglottis* – a small flap of tissue that prevents food and liquid from going into your lungs when you swallow. When you breathe, the epiglottis opens to allow air into your trachea or windpipe, the main airway into your lungs.
- Your right lung has three lobes, and your left lung has two (to accommodate the heart). Each lobe is surrounded by a thin membrane called a *pleura*, which contains a small amount of fluid to prevent friction while you breathe. Another pleura covers each whole lung to prevent friction between your lungs and your chest wall.
- *Bronchi* are the large airways that branch off from your trachea into your lungs. Each bronchus feeds into several smaller airways called bronchioles that reach deep into your lungs, much like a tree spreads out from the main trunk into progressively smaller branches. (Together, the bronchi and bronchioles are often referred to as *bronchial tubes*.)
- Each bronchiole ends in a little bunch of air sacs called *alveoli*, which transfer oxygen into your blood stream and absorb carbon dioxide for you to expel when you exhale.
- Air filtration elements include the hairs in your nose, which trap particles of dust, pollen and other irritants, and the *cilia*, or tiny hairs, that line your bronchial tubes.

The cilia are like little brooms, moving back and forth to sweep mucus out of the airways so you can cough it out. Mucus is like a mop, gathering up irritants and germs to keep them from invading your body.

Your *diaphragm*, the muscle that separates your chest cavity from your abdominal cavity, also is involved in helping you breathe.

Asbestos causes problems because its fibers are extremely fragile and break easily into tiny particles that your body's air filtration system can't trap and expel. The longer you're exposed to asbestos dust, the more likely these fibers are to work their way through your airways and into your body. Even single exposures to small amounts of asbestos can cause mesothelioma. (See Chapter 2 for more details on what asbestos is and what it has been used for.) When asbestos gets into your lungs and stays there, it can cause mesothelioma – which often isn't diagnosed until 10 or more years after your exposure to asbestos dust and particles.

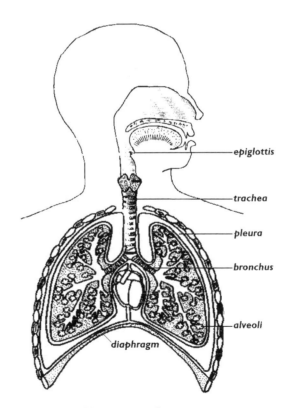

Figure 1-1: Your respiratory system

Types of Mesothelioma

Mesothelioma can be either *benign*, meaning it doesn't grow and spread, or *malignant*, meaning it grows and invades surrounding tissue. Malignant mesothelioma is the most serious of all asbestos-related diseases and can be extremely difficult to diagnose and treat (see Chapter 3).

There are four types of mesothelioma:

- *Pleural mesothelioma* occurs in the membranes, or pleura, surrounding the lungs and the lobes of the lungs. Unlike most cancers, malignant pleural mesothelioma doesn't form a single tumor; instead, it spreads through the pleura like a sheet of water. Symptoms of early-stage mesothelioma are typically quite mild and often lead to misdiagnoses (see Chapter 3). You may experience chronic (ongoing) pain in one area of the chest, weight loss or fever; some patients have difficulty breathing because of fluid build-up that prevents the lungs from expanding freely. Malignant pleural mesothelioma can – and often does – spread to other parts of the body, including the brain.

    Because pleural mesothelioma is difficult to diagnose in its early, more treatable stages and very difficult to treat in its advanced stages, survival rates are low. Fewer than one in ten patients with malignant pleural mesothelioma live three to five years beyond their initial diagnosis.

- *Peritoneal mesothelioma* occurs in the membranes of the abdominal cavity and frequently spreads to the liver, intestines and other organs. Patients with this form of the disease typically report severe abdominal pain, as well as difficulty with bowel movements, nausea and vomiting, swollen feet and fever. One-year survival rates for peritoneal mesothelioma are a bit better than for the pleural variety, but more than half of these patients survive less than a year following the onset of symptoms.

- *Pericardial mesothelioma*, which invades the protective sac that surrounds the heart, makes up only about two percent of all cases of this disease. As the disease progresses, it interferes with the heart's ability to pump oxygen-rich blood through your body, which in turns causes a rapid decline in overall health. Symptoms of pericardial mesothelioma are similar to those of a heart attack: pain in the chest, shortness of breath and nausea.
- *Testicular mesothelioma* attacks the lining of a testicle. Like pericardial mesothelioma, this form of the disease accounts for only about 2 percent of all cases, but it has the best survival rates; more than half of testicular mesothelioma patients live two years or more after their initial diagnosis.

Mesothelioma Stages and Cell Types

Several factors play a role in treating mesothelioma and in survival rates for this disease, including your age and overall health. But two of the most critical factors in determining which treatments are effective are the *stage of the disease* and its *cell type.*

Most forms of cancer are categorized as Stage 0, Stage I, Stage II, Stage III or Stage IV. Stage 0 is cancer that is localized; it hasn't spread to surrounding tissues. Stages I through III indicate more extensive disease; the tumor is large, for example, or cancer cells have spread to nearby lymph nodes and/or organs next to the location of the primary cancer site. Stage IV is cancer that has spread (or *metastasized*) to another organ, typically relatively far from the original cancer site.

> *Depending on your doctor and treatment center, you may run across different staging methods and labels. In general, though, localized mesothelioma is considered Stage 0 or Stage I. Advanced mesothelioma means the cancer has spread.*

Treatment options and survival rates are almost always better when mesothelioma is caught in its early stages. However, because symptoms can easily be mistaken for other ailments (see Chapter 3), mesothelioma often isn't diagnosed until it has progressed to surrounding tissues and organs.

Mesothelioma's cell type, or *histology*, also presents treatment challenges. Some mesothelioma cells come from the lining of membranes, or *epithelial*, layers. These epithelial cancer cells are well-differentiated and have a distinct elongated shape, sort of like mud bricks (see Figure 1-2). Epithelial mesothelioma is the most easily treated and makes up between 50 percent and 75 percent of all mesothelioma diagnoses.

Sarcomatoid mesothelioma involves cells from bone and muscle. These cells are basically oval in shape, but they're more irregular than epithelial cells. Sarcomatoid mesothelioma is less common than the epithelial variety, accounting for between 7 percent and 20 percent of annual diagnoses.

Biphasic mesothelioma includes both epithelial and sarcomatoid cancer cells. Treatment options for both sarcomatoid and biphasic mesothelioma are more challenging because the sarcomatoid cells come from muscle and bone, and it's difficult to destroy the cancerous cells without also damaging or destroying healthy cells. Epithelial mesothelioma also tends to respond better to treatment, so one-year survival rates typically are much better for patients with epithelial mesothelioma.

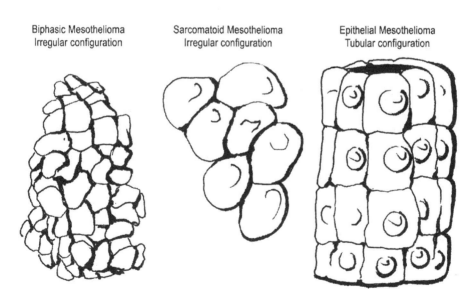

Figure 1-2: Biphasic, sarcomatoid and epithelial mesothelioma cells

Other Asbestos-Related Lung Diseases

Exposure to asbestos can lead to other lung problems besides mesothelioma. Asbestosis is scarring of the lung tissue as a result of inhaling the microscopic fibers in asbestos dust. These fibers can penetrate deep into your lungs and lodge in the tiniest bronchioles and air sacs. When your body detects these foreign invaders, it launches its immune response, deploying specialized cells to try to destroy the fibers. However, because asbestos is resistant to the chemical processes your immune system uses, your body's second defense is to lay down fibrous tissue over the invader to prevent it from spreading. This fibrous tissue eventually encapsulates the asbestos fiber, creating a mass that can obstruct the small airways in your lungs and thicken the walls of the air sacs, which in turn interferes with their ability to infuse your blood with oxygen and remove carbon dioxide. As more of this scar tissue develops, your lungs become unable to expand and contract, and breathing becomes difficult.

About half of all people who are exposed to asbestos over a prolonged period develop *pleural plaques*, localized areas of scar tissue that forms around asbestos fibers. Most pleural plaques are found in the pleura lining the diaphragm (the parietal pleura), but they occasionally occur in the pleura near the ribcage. Unlike asbestosis, pleural plaques apparently stop forming when you're no longer exposed to asbestos. However, depending on your exposure level, pleural plaques also can make breathing difficult – often two decades or more after you were exposed to asbestos.

Pleural plaques are non-cancerous and cannot become malignant. However, patients with pleural plaques often also develop asbestosis or malignant mesothelioma. Nearly all patients with asbestosis, and many with malignant mesothelioma, also have pleural plaques.

Lung cancer – that is, cancer that forms inside the lung tissue, rather than in the lining around the lungs – often goes hand-in-hand with mesothelioma. Although most people associate lung cancer with smoking, nonsmokers who have been exposed to asbestos are as much as six times more likely to develop lung cancer than nonsmokers who have never been exposed to asbestos.

And, just as mesothelioma has a long latency period, asbestos-related lung cancer usually isn't diagnosed until at least 15 years after exposure to asbestos.

Smoking does not increase your risk of developing mesothelioma. However, your doctor will advise quitting smoking to prevent additional damage to your lungs (and most doctors advise quitting regardless of whether you have any lung disease).

Chapter 2

What is Asbestos?

Asbestos is a naturally occurring, heat-resistant mineral that has been used for thousands of years. Archaeologists have found evidence that humans in what is now Finland used asbestos minerals to strengthen cooking pots and utensils 4,500 years ago; the Roman emperor Charlemagne was reputed to have a tablecloth made of asbestos during his reign from 800 to 814; and Marco Polo wrote of being offered clothing that couldn't burn during his travels in Siberia.

Some archaeologists believe that ancient societies made asbestos shrouds for their rulers to prevent their ashes from being mixed with materials from the funeral pyre, and others have found evidence indicating asbestos was used to make "perpetual" wicks for lamps – a practice that continued for centuries. Indeed, the very word asbestos comes from the ancient Greek word for "unquenchable."

In this chapter, learn what asbestos is, how it has been and continues to be used, and how its health hazards were discovered and documented.

Types of Asbestos and Their Uses

Asbestos actually is a set of six minerals. All six asbestos minerals – *actinolite, amosite, anthophyllite, chrysotile, crocidolite and tremolite* – are resistant to heat, fire and damage from chemicals or electricity. Asbestos also absorbs sound, making it useful for such applications as ceiling tile.

Asbestos minerals are composed of very thin, fibrous crystals. Of the six types of asbestos minerals, five are amphibole, or needle-like crystals. Only chrysotile, or white asbestos, crystals are curly (or serpentine). Because of its unique structure, white asbestos is more flexible than its needle-like counterparts and can be woven into fabric.

Although humans have used asbestos sporadically for thousands of years, the mineral came into widespread industrial use in the mid-1800s. In the United States, the first asbestos mine was developed on Staten Island in the late 1850s, and by 1866, asbestos was in common use as insulation in the U.S. and Canada. Less than 100 years later, asbestos was common in concrete, bricks, fireplace mortar, pipes, and fire-retardant coatings.

About 95 percent of all asbestos-containing materials in U.S. buildings are made with white asbestos, which has been used in the following ways:

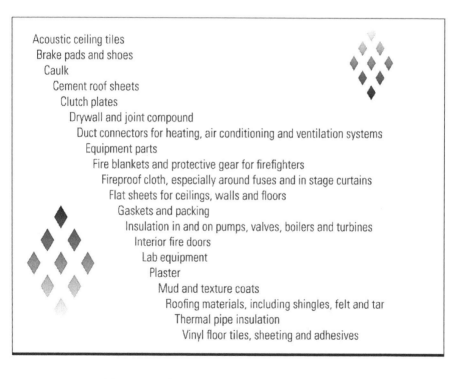

Figure 1-3: Uses of Asbestos Chart

Amosite, also known as brown asbestos, is the second most common type of asbestos found in U.S. buildings. Although most developed countries banned all forms of amphibole, or needle-like, asbestos by the mid-1990s, products containing these kinds of asbestos still can be found in many structures. Such products include:

- Low-density insulating board and ceiling tiles
- Asbestos-reinforced cement sheets and pipes used in construction and casings for water, electrical and telecommunications systems
- Thermal and chemical insulation

Over the years, asbestos found its way into far more than just building supplies and car parts. At one point, artificial Christmas snow, or flocking, was made with asbestos. Kent brand cigarettes used asbestos in its filters in the 1950s. And before the 1960s, gas mask filters contained asbestos. Other filters, including those used to remove particulates from chemical compounds and even wine, also were made with asbestos. It was even used in lawn furniture and some art supplies.

Asbestos also can contaminate other minerals. For example, the mineral vermiculite, which has been used as an asbestos substitute, sometimes contains small amounts of asbestos. One vermiculite mine in Libby, Montana, was contaminated and the Environmental Protection Agency has designated it a Superfund clean-up area.

In 2000, lab tests showed asbestos contamination in major brands of crayons, including Crayola. The asbestos was believed to have contaminated the industrial-grade talc the manufacturers used to make their crayons, and, as a result of the tests, all U.S. crayon manufacturers removed talc from their formulations.

Discovery of the Health Hazards of Asbestos

The nature of asbestos makes it especially easy to inhale. Asbestos fibers are extremely fragile and can break into tiny particles that are invisible to the naked eye, and activities like mixing, cutting, scraping, and even sweeping can make the particles airborne.

Although different types of asbestos have different chemical properties, all types are now known to be harmful to human health. Since at least the early 1900s, when researchers noticed a large number of lung problems and early deaths in asbestos mining towns, physicians and public health officials have investigated the impacts of asbestos. Many companies failed to do any research to determine whether asbestos was harmful. Other companies knew of its dangers but hid that knowledge from workers and their families.

The following timeline highlights some of the more important discoveries and documentation regarding the toxicity of asbestos.

Asbestos-Related Dangers Timeline

Year	Event
1898	Annual report of Britain's Chief Inspector of Factories notes that asbestos has "easily demonstrated" health risks.
1906	First documented asbestos-related death.
1918	A U.S. study notes that "in the practice of American and Canadian life insurance companies, asbestos workers are generally declined on account of the assumed health-injurious conditions of the industry."
1924	First diagnosis of asbestosis (see Chapter 3).
1927	First known U.S worker's compensation claim for asbestos-related disease.
Late 1920s	A large public health study, generally known as the Merewether Report (named after one of its authors), found that about 25 percent of examined British asbestos-textile workers suffered from lung disease, leading to stronger regulation of asbestos-related manufacturing.
1931	The term *mesothelioma* makes its first appearance in the medical literature.
1932	In a letter to an asbestos manufacturer, the U.S. Bureau of Mines notes that "asbestos dust is one of the most dangerous dusts to which man is exposed."

Asbestos-Related Dangers Timeline

Year	Event
1934	Officials of two major asbestos companies edit an article about diseases in asbestos workers to minimize the reported dangers of asbestos dust.
1936	A group of asbestos companies sponsored research on the health effects of asbestos dust, but refused to allow the research findings to be published without their approval.
1944	A report by Metropolitan Life Insurance Company finds that more than 20 percent of a group of 195 asbestos miners suffer from asbestosis (see Chapter 3).
1951	Asbestos companies deleted all references to cancer in research they had sponsored before agreeing to publication of the research findings.
1953	Officials at National Gypsum prevent delivery of a letter the company's safety director had written to the Indiana Division of Industrial Hygiene. The safety director had recommended that workers mixing acoustic plaster wear respirators because of the product's asbestos content.
1953	Mesothelioma is reported in an asbestos insulator.
1955	A major epidemiological study demonstrates that asbestos workers have a tenfold risk above the general population of contracting lung cancer.
1960	Another epidemiological study confirms reports that exposure to asbestos causes mesothelioma. This study also included the children and wives of asbestos workers who contracted mesothelioma.

Asbestos-Related Dangers Timeline

Year	Event
1964	Dr. Irving Selikoff, a major researcher at Mt. Sinai Hospital in New York, confirms widespread disease among asbestos workers and from family members living with asbestos workers. A large number of job titles were implicated in the report, including construction workers, electricians, plumbers, and carpenters. Selikoff pointed out that asbestos did not "respect" job titles and could harm any person who breathed in asbestos.
Late 1960s	After 1964, the medical literature continued to identify asbestos as a major carcinogen and environmental hazard. Over 200 publications described the hazards of asbestos by the end of the 1960's.
Late 1970s	The U.S. Consumer Product Safety Commission bans the use of asbestos in gas fireplaces and wallboard patching materials because using them can release asbestos into the air.
1979	Electric hairdryer manufacturers voluntarily stop using asbestos in their products.
1980s	The Health Effects Institute in Cambridge, Massachusetts begins evaluating the lifetime cancer risks of people who work and live in buildings with asbestos products, as well as the risk of service workers in such buildings.
1989	The Environmental Protection Agency issues the Asbestos Ban and Phase Out Rule. The rule is subsequently thrown out by a federal appeals court, so uses developed before 1989 are still legal in the U.S. Asbestos is still not banned in the U.S.

Asbestos-Related Dangers Timeline

Year	Event
2000	Although the Consumer Product Safety Commission concludes that the risk posed by asbestos fibers in crayons is low, U.S. crayon manufactures agree to stop using talc in their products.
2000	The Environmental Protection Agency determines that asbestos-contaminated vermiculite poses a risk and recommends that consumers take measures to reduce dust generation when working with vermiculite, such as making it damp, using it in well-ventilated areas, and using premixed potting soil.

Dr. Barry Castleman's book, *Asbestos: Medical and Legal Aspects*, is an excellent resource on the history of discoveries and knowledge about asbestos and its dangers. Dr. Castleman has spent years researching and documenting the wrongdoing of asbestos companies.

Chapter 3

Diagnosing Mesothelioma

Diagnosing mesothelioma, especially in its early stages, is difficult because its symptoms are similar to many other kinds of illness. For example, one of the most common symptoms is shortness of breath, which also can be caused by such things as asthma and other lung ailments, and heart disease, as well as various forms of cancer.

This chapter covers the common symptoms associated with mesothelioma and other asbestos-related diseases, as well as various tests your doctor may order to make a diagnosis.

Mesothelioma Symptoms

Especially in early-stage mesothelioma, symptoms often are non-specific, meaning they can be caused by a number of things. Only a handful of mesothelioma patients have no symptoms at all. Most patients experience one or more of the following symptoms:

- Shortness of breath, with or without chest pain
- Pleural effusions (which may feel like pressure on the chest or abdomen)
- Chest or back pain, especially noticeable on one side
- Abdominal pain or swelling
- Unexplained weight loss, loss of appetite, fever or muscle weakness

Keeping track of your symptoms is key to helping your doctor diagnose your illness and evaluate your treatment (see Chapter 4). Use the personal medical journal in the back of this book (Appendix B) to track your symptoms and their severity.

> *If you have any of these symptoms, talk with your doctor right away. Your survival chances improve with early detection and diagnosis. Make sure you tell your doctor about any known asbestos exposure and any occupational risk factors (see Chapter 2) so he or she knows to check for mesothelioma.*

The following sections describe common mesothelioma symptoms in more detail.

Shortness of Breath

It's normal to feel short of breath when you're exercising or doing something strenuous, such as moving or carrying something heavy. But shortness of breath (called *dyspnea*) can indicate disease when you experience it during activities that normally wouldn't cause any breathing symptoms, such as doing household chores, climbing stairs, or walking at a leisurely pace. Be sure to tell your doctor if you start getting short of breath during activities that you've been accustomed to doing without problems.

Shortness of breath is a subjective symptom, so your doctor will ask several questions to determine whether it's cause for concern. He or she will ask you to describe how you feel physically when you get short of breath and whether you experience any pain in the chest or back. Other symptoms that often accompany shortness of breath—and that may indicate problems other than mesothelioma—include palpitations, wheezing, and coughing.

Pleural Effusion

Pleural effusion is another common symptom associated with asbestos exposure. Pleural effusion is a build-up of fluid in the pleura. Normally, the tiny blood vessels in the pleura produce lubricating fluid that allows the two sides of the pleura to glide smoothly against one another. Extra fluid is usually carried away by the blood vessels and lymph system.

When something goes wrong – either too much fluid is produced or excess fluid isn't carried away – the pleura can't move properly and you experience shortness of breath, often accompanied by pain or a heavy sensation in the chest.

As with shortness of breath, lots of health conditions can cause pleural effusion, including asbestos exposure and its related diseases. Pleural effusion is common with pleural plaque, asbestosis and malignant mesothelioma, but it doesn't indicate asbestos-related diseases by itself; your doctor will have to perform several tests to diagnose the underlying cause of the effusion.

Chest or Back Pain

More than half of mesothelioma patients experience pain in one side of the chest or back. This pain usually is caused by pleural effusion, and it's rare to have pleural effusion in both lungs.

Abdominal Pain or Swelling

When fluid builds up in the lining of the abdominal cavity (*the peritoneal pleura*), you may experience swelling, pressure, or pain. This symptom is more common with peritoneal mesothelioma than with pleural mesothelioma, but it also can indicate either a spreading of the cancer or other health issues.

Unexplained Weight Loss

About a third of mesothelioma patients experience unexplained weight loss. This symptom is more common in patients with peritoneal mesothelioma (see Chapter 1) but occasionally occurs with pleural mesothelioma. Unexplained weight loss also may be accompanied by abdominal pain, bowel obstruction (again, more common in peritoneal mesothelioma), nausea and loss of appetite, and anemia.

Other Symptoms

Mesothelioma patients sometimes experience other symptoms, although these other symptoms aren't as common as those listed above. For example, a few (less than 1 percent) patients experience difficulty swallowing, chronic hoarseness, and coughing up blood.

Some patients also experience fever, muscle weakness, and numbness (or sensory loss). Swelling in the face or neck can indicate that the cancer has spread beyond the mesothelium.

Patients with peritoneal mesothelioma may have bowel obstructions, caused by a tumor pressing on the organs in the abdomen. Peritoneal mesothelioma also can cause increased frequency of urination, loss of muscle tissue, fever, and night sweats.

Diagnosing Mesothelioma

As with many other diseases, early detection of mesothelioma greatly improves your long-term survival chances and may give you more treatment options. However, because mesothelioma's symptoms are similar to many other diseases, your doctor likely will conduct a number of tests to rule out other causes and confirm a mesothelioma diagnosis. During the initial evaluation of your symptoms, your doctor will talk to you about your asbestos exposure or risk and your own and your family's medical history to decide which tests to order.

He or she will listen to your lungs and chest cavity and may conduct *spirometry* or lung function tests. Spirometry tests reveal how well you're able to take in and expel air. You place your lips tightly around the mouthpiece and take as deep a breath as you can, then exhale as forcefully as you can for as long as you can. You may repeat this procedure three or more times to ensure a correct reading. Results depend on a number of factors, including age, sex, ethnicity and general health; your results will be compared with normal (or "expected") results for your demographic group.

Based on your initial exam, your doctor will order one or more imaging tests to get a look inside your chest and/or abdominal cavity. Imaging tests are useful both for diagnosing your disease and for developing a treatment plan and tracking your body's response to treatment, so you'll likely undergo several imaging tests during your treatment.

Imaging Tests

X-rays are the most common and least expensive imaging tests, but they often don't provide enough detail to diagnose mesothelioma. So your doctor may order one of the following:

- *CT scan.* CT (*computed tomography*) scans use x-rays and computers to draw more detailed pictures of your internal organs.
- *MRI.* MRI (*magnetic resonance imaging*) uses a magnetic field and radio waves to scan your body. MRI scans provide a much clearer picture of soft tissue than CT scans and sometimes are used to confirm a diagnosis based on a CT scan. MRI also is very useful for determining the stage of disease and planning surgical procedures.
- *PET scan.* PET (*positron emission tomography*) scans measure functional activity in your body. They're used most often to determine whether cancer has spread far from its point of origin.
- *PET-CT scan.* This machine combines CT and PET technology and can provide your doctor with a better overall picture of your physical health.

The following sections describe these tests, what to expect, and how to prepare for them in more detail.

X-Ray

X-ray machines generate a tiny burst of radiation (generally recognized as safe) that passes through your body and records an image of your bones and internal organs on a special plate.

Chest x-rays are inexpensive and are often used as a preliminary imaging test when your doctor suspects mesothelioma or wants to rule out other lung diseases like emphysema or lung cancer. Many doctors' offices have their own x-ray machines, or you may be referred to an imaging facility or hospital for the test. Chest x-rays generally don't require anything in the way of preparation, and you won't experience any pain or side effects. If you have trouble standing, you may be able to sit or lie down during the x-ray.

You undress from the waist up and put on an exam gown. You also need to remove any jewelry that may obscure the x-ray image, such as necklaces and earrings. You also may be asked to remove eyeglasses.

During the x-ray, a technician positions your body between the camera and the plate. For a front view, you stand against the plate, holding your arms up or at your sides and rolling your shoulders forward to allow for a better image of your lungs. You take a deep breath and hold it for a few seconds while the image is taken (inhaling or exhaling during the x-ray can blur the image). Holding an inhaled breath inflates your lungs and provides a better image.

The technician also may take side views, where you stand with one shoulder against the plate and raise your arms over your head. Again, you take a deep breath and hold it while the technician takes the image.

Your doctor and/or a radiologist examine the x-rays to see what's going on in your lungs. Early-stage mesothelioma is difficult to detect on x-rays, and pleural thickening, which often occurs in later-stage lung disease, can hide the signs of mesothelioma. However, pleural effusions are often seen on x-rays and are a key indicator of mesothelioma.

CT Scan

CT machines take x-rays from several angles, and computer software manipulates the images to create cross-sectional views of your bones and soft tissues. Depending on the machine, the CT technician can even create three-dimensional images from the x-rays. Few clinics or doctors' offices have their own CT machines, so you'll go to an imaging center or hospital for this test.

CT machines look like long tubes with an opening in the middle. You lie on a narrow table that slides in and out of the machine, and the machine rotates around you to take x-rays at different angles. You have to lie still -- with your arms either at your side or stretched out over your head -- during the scan to prevent the images from being blurred. The technician may use pillows or straps to keep you in the proper position, and some people experience feelings of claustrophobia in a CT machine.

You'll be asked to undress and put on an exam gown, and you'll remove any jewelry so it doesn't interfere with the imaging. For most CTs, you'll be told not to eat anything for several hours before the scan. Depending on what your doctor is looking for, you may have to drink a preparation of *contrast material* – a special dye that provides sharper images by highlighting or outlining certain parts of your body. You also may have contrast material injected into a vein in your arm.

> *Some people have allergic reactions to the contrast material. Usually these reactions are minor, such as hives and a small itchy rash around the injection site. But, although rare, some people have severe reactions that can be life-threatening. Be sure to tell your doctor about any allergies you have and what reactions you had if you've been given contrast material before.*

When the technician is ready to begin the scan, he or she will go into a separate room. You'll communicate with each other through an intercom. You'll hear some clicking and whirring noises while the machine takes the images. As we mentioned, some people feel claustrophobic in a CT machine and your position may not feel comfortable, but the scan itself is painless and relatively brief. As with chest x-rays, you may be asked to hold your breath for a few seconds to ensure that the images aren't blurred.

After the CT scan, you'll be able to return to your normal routine. If you were given contrast material, you may be asked to stay at the facility for a while to ensure you aren't suffering any ill effects from the dye, and you may receive some special instructions for after you leave. Generally, if you've been given contrast material, you'll be advised to drink lots of water to help your kidneys flush the dye out of your system.

A radiologist will look at the CT images on a computer screen and send a report to your doctor. Because of the improved detail of the CT, the radiologist can identify small tumors and abnormal build-up of fluids (effusions). CT images also can help your doctor pinpoint the best place to get a biopsy (covered later in this chapter), and can help show whether and how far any cancer has spread.

MRI

MRI machines look similar to CT machines, except they use a strong magnetic field and radio waves to create detailed images of your body. The magnetic field aligns the water molecules in your body, and the radio waves generate faint signals from those molecules to produce cross-sectional images of bones, organs, and soft tissue.

Because MRI uses a magnetic field, any metal in your body can affect both the image and your safety. Tell your doctor and the MRI technologist if you have:

- *A pacemaker*
- *An implanted heart defibrillator*
- *Artificial heart valves*
- *Metallic joint replacements*
- *Cochlear (ear) implants*
- *Metal clips (used to prevent aneurysms from leaking)*
- *Shrapnel, bullet or any other kind of metal fragment in your body*

Also tell your doctor and the MRI technologist about any kidney or liver problems you may have. Certain kidney and liver issues may require changes or limits on using injected contrast materials (see the CT section earlier in this chapter).

Unless your doctor tells you otherwise, you can eat and drink normally before your MRI. You'll change into an exam gown and remove any jewelry, watches, hairpins, eyeglasses, wigs, dentures, and hearing aids. Women will have to remove their bras, especially those with underwires.

As with the CT scan, you'll lie on a narrow table that moves in and out of the MRI machine and will communicate with the technologist via an intercom. The MRI scan is painless but noisy; the machine makes repetitive thumping, tapping, and other sounds. You may wear earplugs or listen to music on headphones to help block the noise. Some people feel claustrophobic in an MRI machine; if your claustrophia is severe, talk to your doctor about taking a sedative before the scan.

MRIs also require you to remain still while the images are taken, and you may be given contrast materials to enhance the appearance of certain tissues and organs.

If you haven't been sedated, you can resume your normal routine immediately after the scan. If you've been given contrast materials, you should drink plenty of water to help flush those materials from your body.

A radiologist reads the MRI images and compares them to any chest x-rays or CT scans you've had, then sends a report to your doctor, who will share the results with you.

PET Scans

X-rays, CT scans, and MRIs look at your bones and internal organs as whole structures. PET scans look at the activity of the cells inside your body. They can be particularly useful in detecting mesothelioma and certain other types of cancer. For a PET scan, you'll be injected with a radioactive glucose (sugar) solution, and you may experience a cold sensation moving up your arm from the injection site. (Sometimes patients inhale or swallow the solution, but injection into a vein is most common.) Cancer cells use more energy than normal cells, so they pull in the glucose at a higher rate than normal cells do. The radioactive component of the solution causes cancer cells to show up as bright spots on the scan images.

The glucose solution raises your blood sugar levels, so you'll be given specific instructions on what you can eat and drink in the 24 hours before your scan. Generally, you won't eat or drink anything (except water) for at least four to six hours before the scan. When you arrive at the imaging facility or hospital, you'll receive the glucose injection, and then you'll lie quietly for about an hour to give the solution time to circulate throughout your body. The scan itself lasts for between 15 and 30 minutes, and, as with other imaging tests, you'll have to lie very still to ensure the images aren't blurred.

Before your scan, you should talk with your doctor about all medications you take, including any over-the-counter drugs, vitamins, dietary supplements, and herbal preparations. You also should avoid strenuous physical activity in the 24 hours before your scan. It's critical that you follow your doctor's pre-scan instructions closely to avoid potential problems with the quality of the images and possible complications from the glucose solution.

Most PET scan facilities also recommend that you wear warm, comfortable clothing the day of your scan, because the scanner rooms often are kept at cooler-than-normal temperatures. You may be asked to change into an exam gown before the scan. You'll also go to the bathroom to empty your bladder before your scan, and, if an area near your bladder needs to be examined, you may have a catheter to keep your bladder drained during the scan.

PET scan machines are similar in design to CT and MRI machines; see the descriptions in those sections earlier in this chapter. The PET machine makes buzzing and clicking sounds, similar to a CT machine but not as loud as an MRI.

After the scan, you should be able to resume your normal routine, but you'll want to drink plenty of water afterwards to help flush the radioactive solution from your body.

A radiologist trained in reading PET scans will interpret the results and report them to your doctor, who will discuss them with you.

PET-CT Scans

Combination PET-CT scans provide the most clarity of any current imaging tests, by combining the CT's view of the structure of your body's bones, organs, and soft tissues with the PET's detection of activity at the cellular level. Cellular changes can show up long before any structural changes – such as tumors – appear, making this particular test very useful in diagnosing certain diseases, locating the source of cancer and any places where it may have spread, and tracking how well treatment is working (see Chapter 4).

Taking Biopsies

Imaging tests can help your doctor pinpoint potential disease, but none of the imaging tests discussed in this chapter can definitively diagnose mesothelioma. To confirm the diagnosis, your doctor probably will order a *biopsy*, in which a sample of tissue or fluid is removed and examined.

Before a biopsy is taken and tested, your doctor likely will refer to a *mass*, *lesion* or other nonspecific term – instead of "tumor," for example – as a subtle reminder that, until the biopsy is complete, neither you nor your doctor can know for sure what it is. Biopsies most frequently are used to determine whether an abnormal area of tissue or fluid is cancerous, but these tests also can be used to identify other conditions, such as infections and certain autoimmune diseases (such as lupus).

When the sample tissue or fluid is collected, it's usually sent to a lab where a *pathologist* – a doctor who specializes in identifying and studying the nature, causes, and progression of disease –

prepares the sample with special solutions and applies certain dyes, called *immunostains*, to make abnormal cells stand out under a microscope.

The pathologist examines these abnormal cells to determine whether you have cancer and, if so, what type. Preliminary biopsy results can take as little as a few minutes, but complete examination of the sample usually takes a week or two. Sometimes, the sample is sent to a second hospital or lab, where another pathologist reviews the results. The pathologist also will determine the cell type of any mesothelioma: epithelial, sarcomatoid, or biphasic (see Chapter 1).

For mesothelioma patients, there are two main types of biopsy procedure: noninvasive, often called *needle biopsies*, and *surgical biopsies*. The following sections offer more detail on these procedures.

Needle Biopsies

Needle biopsies are less invasive than surgical biopsies because they don't involve incisions and usually don't involve general anaesthesia. You'll receive a local anaesthetic to numb the area where the needle is inserted, and your doctor may give you pain medications to take after the biopsy to minimize any discomfort. For most patients, post-biopsy pain and soreness last only a few days. Pain during the procedure typically is low, and most patients experience only a sense of increased pressure when the needle is inserted. The doctor may insert and withdraw the needle several times to ensure enough cells are collected.

Sometimes doctors order image-guided biopsies, using ultrasound or CT machines to pinpoint the proper site from which to take the sample.

Needle biopsies usually are performed in a hospital or outpatient surgical facility. In some cases, your doctor may ask you to avoid eating or drinking for several hours before the procedure; in other cases, fasting won't be necessary. If you're on blood thinners or certain other medications, your doctor may tell you to stop taking them a few days before and after the biopsy to reduce the risk of internal bleeding. Ask your doctor for specific instructions and follow them carefully to avoid complications.

After the sample is collected, your health care team will dress the insertion site with a bandage; you may be asked to hold it in place, applying some pressure for a few minutes to minimize bleeding. You may stay in a quiet room for a while until any anaesthesia or sedatives wear off, or you may be kept for several hours for observation to ensure there aren't any complications.

If you're sedated or under general anaesthesia for your biopsy, you won't be able to drive or return to work after the procedure. You should make arrangements with family members or friends to drive you home, stay with you for 24 hours, and help with domestic chores for a day or two.

Mesothelioma patients typically have one of the following needle biopsy procedures:

- *Pleural biopsy.* A needle is used to take fluid and tissue samples from the chest and pleural membrane.

- *Thoracentesis.* This is usually ordered for patients who have excessive fluid built up in the chest cavity. Thoracentesis both collects samples for testing and drains excess fluid to help make the patient more comfortable.

- *Paracentesis.* Patients with peritoneal mesothelioma (see Chapter 1) often experience excess fluid build-up in the abdominal cavity. Paracentesis, like thoracentesis for pleural mesothelioma, is used to drain the excess fluid and collect samples for testing and diagnosis.

Cytology is when fluid only (not tissue) is collected. Fluid itself, however, may not provide a definitive diagnosis. If the fluid sample is negative, it means there are no cancer cells in the fluid – but it doesn't mean there are no cancer cells in the tissues.

Surgical Biopsies

Surgical biopsies for mesothelioma involve cutting into the chest or abdomen to remove either a larger sample of tissue (called an *incisional biopsy*) or an entire suspicious mass (an *excisional biopsy*). Surgical biopsies usually are ordered when the target area can't be reached by needle or when the samples collected from a needle biopsy don't yield conclusive test results. Again, fluid may not provide a definitive diagnosis, so a tissue sample may be required.

You may have local or general anesthesia for a surgical biopsy, depending on where the target sample is located. You also may have to stay in the hospital for observation for a few hours, or even overnight, after a surgical biopsy.

The most common surgical biopsy procedures for mesothelioma are:

- *Thoracoscopy/thoracotomy.* A thoracoscope looks a bit like a long, thin telescope. It's attached to a video camera and is inserted through a small incision in the chest. *Thorascopy* refers to using the scope to examine the pleura and other areas of the chest; *thoracotomy* means taking samples of the pleura or pericardial mesothelium to test for mesothelioma (see Chapter 1). A thorascopy is often referred to as *VATS*, for *video assisted thoracic surgery* (see Chapter 4).

- *Laparoscopy/laparotomy.* This procedure is similar to thoracoscopy, except that the incision is made in the abdomen and the scope is used to view and take samples of peritoneal tissue.

- *Mediastinoscopy.* To view lymph nodes and take samples, the scope is inserted under the *sternum* (breast bone) at the neck. This procedure is often used to help your doctor diagnose mesothelioma and determine how advanced it is. When a mesothelioma patient's lymph nodes test positive for cancer, it means that the disease has progressed at least to Stage 3 (see Chapter 1).

Testing for and diagnosing mesothelioma can feel like a long process. But adequate testing is essential to confirm the disease and how advanced it is, and you and your doctor can't come up with a sensible treatment plan until you know exactly what you're dealing with. Turn to Chapter 4 to learn about various treatment options.

Chapter 4

Treating Mesothelioma

A mesothelioma diagnosis can be devastating. However, while there is no cure for mesothelioma – that is, no way to permanently eliminate the disease – you can undergo treatments that can help slow the progress of the disease and ease the severity of your symptoms.

Even though there is no cure, with mesothelioma, as with most serious diseases, treatment strategies are referred to as either curative or palliative in intent. Curative treatments attempt to cure or control the disease, while palliative treatments are aimed at reducing symptoms and making the patient more comfortable. The earlier mesothelioma is detected and diagnosed, the more successful curative strategies tend to be. However, it's not uncommon to begin your treatment with curative strategies and move to palliative treatments later on.

The treatment plan you and your doctor develop depends on several factors, including the type and stage of disease and your overall health. Conventional mesothelioma treatment plans generally include chemotherapy, radiation and surgery – or, most commonly, a combination of these methods (called *multimodal treatment*). Less conventional treatments include experimental options such as gene therapy. Alternative medicine offers some unique benefits to improve your general sense of well-being and even counteract some of the side effects of conventional treatments; learn more about these options in Chapter 5.

This chapter walks you through your conventional treatment options, showing you the pros and cons and what you can expect from each. And, because choosing the right doctor and treatment facility is critical to the success of your treatment plan, the final section of this chapter is devoted to this topic.

Surgery

Surgery may be used to diagnose mesothelioma and determine the stage or to extend your life by removing tumors that are causing pain or other symptoms (called palliative surgery). Unless mesothelioma is diagnosed in its early stages, surgery may not be an option.

Diagnostic surgery

Your *thorax* is the upper part of your torso. The *thoracic cavity* is the area of your torso from your neck to your diaphragm (see Chapter 1) that contains your heart and lungs. Thus, any surgery involving your thoracic cavity is called *thoracic surgery*.

Surgeons use one of two main techniques for thoracic surgery:

- *Thoracotomy.* In a thoracotomy, the surgeon makes a large incision in the chest wall to gain access to the heart, lungs, and diaphragm. Where the incision is made depends on the type of surgery being performed. For most mesothelioma patients, the incision will be along the ribcage on the side of the affected lung.

- *Video-assisted thoracic surgery (VATS).* In VATS, the surgeon makes a small incision and uses a tiny camera connected to a monitor to view the interior of the thoracic cavity. VATS is less invasive because it causes less damage to the muscle surrounding the chest cavity. However, some surgeries require the larger incision of a thoracotomy to remove damaged tissues and organs.

Life-Extending Surgery

The goal of curative surgery is to remove all visible traces of disease – called a ***macroscopically complete resection***. *Resection* is the surgical removal of all or part of an organ, specific tissue or structure. *Macroscopic* means visible to the naked eye.

If you are a candidate for curative surgery, you'll undergo one of two procedures: *pluerectomy/decortication* or *extraplueral pneumonectomy*. Both of these surgeries are considered radical because they're highly invasive and involve significant recovery time. However, they are known to extend the life of patients with early-stage mesothelioma.

> We strongly believe that these surgeries should be performed by recommended surgeons at mesothelioma treatment centers (see Appendix A).

The following sections describe these procedures in more detail.

Pleurectomy/Decortication

Pleurectomy means removing the pleura. *Decortication* means removing the layer of fibrous tissue surrounding the lung; when this tissue is damaged, it can restrict the lung's ability to expand when you inhale.

A *pleurectomy/decortication (or PD)* surgery involves cutting through the chest wall on the side of the affected lung and pleura and spreading the ribs apart (occasionally the surgeon will remove one rib to gain better access to the chest cavity), then removing the pleura and peeling away the fibrous layer around the lung. In some cases, the surgeon also will remove the pericardium (see Chapter 1) and the diaphragm, and will likely take lymph nodes from the chest cavity so they can be tested for signs of cancer and to help identify the stage of the disease. The results of the lymph node tests will be used to guide the rest of your treatment plan.

If the surgeon removes the diaphragm or pericardium, he or she will replace it with a mesh material designed to imitate the function of the original tissue. Several drainage tubes will be inserted to prevent fluid build-up. After surgery, the patient typically spends a few days in the intensive care unit to ensure there are no complications, then embarks on a rehabilitation program to restore muscle movement and lung function.

> *Pleurectomy/decortication is a highly invasive procedure and requires a lengthy recovery period. Even without complications, you should expect that it will be some time before you feel completely recovered from the operation.*

The most common complications with this procedure involve blood loss, problems with reconstructing the diaphragm and pericardium, and breathing problems associated with manipulating the lung during the surgery. However, surgeons know what to watch for and how to deal with these complications, and most feel that the operation is worth it for patients with early-stage mesothelioma because it maximizes your odds of long-term survival.

Extrapleural Pneumonectomy

An *extrapleural pneumonectomy (or EPP)* is similar to the pleurectomy/decortication procedure described above, but in an EPP, the surgeon also removes the affected lung – and possibly the diaphragm. EPPs are done when the mesothelioma has spread beyond the pleura and has begun infiltrating the lung, or when asbestos-related lung cancer is present in addition to mesothelioma.

In many cases, a surgeon goes into the procedure expecting to perform a pleurectomy but finds that the imaging tests (see Chapter 3) didn't accurately reveal the extent of the disease. (The opposite also can happen but is more rare.) In these cases, an EPP may be performed.

Because mesothelioma is most often diagnosed after it has spread, EPP was a fairly common procedure. However, recent studies have shown that pleurectomies are as effective as EPPs in extending patients' lives. Pleurectomies also have the advantage of saving your lung.

Complications can be more severe than with a pleurectomy, but experienced surgeons are aware of the potential complications and can make adjustments as needed.

Although not every patient is a good candidate for EPP, those who are – and who undergo other forms of treatment in combination with the surgery – tend to have longer survival times than those who opt not to have the surgery.

> *Tip: Dr. Harvey Pass at New York University is a leading surgeon for mesothelioma patients. See his entry in Appendix A (page 109).*

Palliative Surgeries

Not all surgeries are intended to treat the disease itself. Some are intended to relieve symptoms and improve the patient's quality of life. Palliative surgeries for mesothelioma reduce fluid build-up or pressure that makes it difficult to breathe. They don't affect the progress of the disease itself, but – combined with other treatments – they can lessen your symptoms and make you feel better.

The most common palliative surgeries for mesothelioma are:

- *Debulking pleurectomy.* In a debulking pleurectomy, the surgeon removes as much of the cancer from the pleura as possible to ease the pressure on the lungs. This procedure is often combined with *pleurodesis* (see the next bullet) to make breathing easier and improve the patient's quality of life.

- *Pleurodesis.* In this procedure, the surgeon fuses the pleura lining the lungs with the parietal pleura surrounding the chest wall and diaphragm. Fusing these pleura together prevents fluid build-up and pleural effusions (see Chapter 1). Pleurodesis is the most common palliative surgery for mesothelioma patients.

> *Consider all your options before you decide to have a pleurodesis performed. This procedure may make it impossible for you to have a pleurectomy later on should you need it.*

- *Decortication.* Decortication is a procedure in which the surgeon strips away the layer of fibrous tissue surrounding the lung. When this fibrous tissue is damaged, it loses its elasticity and keeps the lung from inflating fully when you inhale. Removing this layer allows the lung to expand better. Decortication sometimes is performed along with pleurodesis to ease symptoms.

- *Catheters and shunts.* Patients who have late-stage mesothelioma and don't want to undergo more invasive treatments sometimes choose to have catheters or shunts implanted to relieve the symptoms of fluid build-up in the pleura surrounding the lungs or abdomen.

> *Palliative surgeries are designed to help relieve symptoms and make you more comfortable. They don't cure your disease or stop or slow down the progress of mesothelioma.*

Chemotherapy

Chemotherapy is the most common treatment for mesothelioma because, most of the time, the disease is already in its later stages (see Chapter 1) by the time it's diagnosed. **Chemotherapy** is the use of chemicals to destroy cancerous cells. Normal cells have complex regulatory structures that control how quickly they grow and how often they divide. When they grow or divide too fast, these regulatory mechanisms force cells to commit suicide, a process called *apoptosis*. In cancer cells, the normal regulatory mechanisms break down, so these cells grow and divide uncontrollably. Chemotherapy drugs are designed to interfere with the process that drives this out-of-control growth.

Unfortunately, chemotherapy drugs don't distinguish between cancerous and normal cells, so they kill off healthy cells as well. Most chemo drugs target rapidly dividing cells, because this is a hallmark of cancerous cells. But some normal cells in your body divide rapidly, too – particularly cells in your bone marrow that generate new red blood cells, the cells that line your stomach and intestines, and the cells in your hair follicles that generate new hair growth. Because most chemo drugs can't differentiate between healthy fast-dividing cells and cancerous cells, patients who undergo chemotherapy commonly experience anemia, nausea or other digestive disruption, and hair loss.

Some of these side effects can be controlled with medication, and researchers are working on identifying specific portals in cancer cells (which aren't present in healthy cells) that would allow the chemicals to penetrate and kill off cancer cells without affecting normal cells. At present, though, chemotherapy is still an imperfect treatment.

The most common chemo treatment for mesothelioma is the combination of **Alimta (pemetrexed),** which was approved by the U.S. Food & Drug Administration in 2004, and **cisplatin**, a longstanding staple of many chemo treatments. More information about each of these drugs is in the following sections, which provide details on different types of chemo drugs, when chemotherapy is used, and how it's used.

Types of Chemotherapy Drugs

In general, chemotherapy drugs are divided into four types or classes, depending on the mechanism they use to kill off cancer cells:

- *Antifolates.* Folic acid, or folate, is a crucial component of cell growth and division; the DNA in cells needs folic acid to replicate itself and generate a new cell. **Antifolate** drugs inhibit cell growth and division by interfering with DNA replication. Antifolates are part of a larger class of drugs known as **antimetabolites,** which work by fooling cells into thinking they're the substances the cells need to grow and divide. But these drugs have important differences that inhibit rather than encourage **cell metabolism,** the chemical processes cells use to function and reproduce. In the case of antifolates, for example, cells take in the drug and attempt to use it help to replicate DNA, but because the drug isn't really folic acid, the replication process breaks down.

Antifolates are believed to work with mesothelioma because this particular type of cancer cell has a high number of receptors that are tuned to taking in folic acid. Because of the higher number of these receptors, mesothelioma cells are more susceptible to being "fooled" into taking in antifolate drugs instead of actual folic acid.

Pemetrexed (also known as Alimta) is an antifolate drug commonly used in mesothelioma chemo treatments. This drug slows the growth and spread of cancer cells and is effective at decreasing pain and extending the lifespan of cancer patients. About 80 percent of mesothelioma patients who undergo chemotherapy take pemetrexed with cisplatin (see the next section). This combination has shown good results in extending mesothelioma patients' lives.

- *Platinum agents.* Platinum agents attack a cell's DNA and disrupt its structure, thus triggering the cell's pre-programmed "suicide" response (apoptosis). Cisplatin is the oldest of the chemo platinum agents and is still considered the standard (in combination with pemetrexed) for mesothelioma chemotherapy. Other platinum agents include *carboplatin* and *oxaliplatin*. If a patient has trouble tolerating cisplatin, which has significant side effects in some patients, carboplatin may be used as a substitute in mesothelioma treatment.

- *Anthracyclines.* Anthracyclines damage a cell's DNA and thus interfere with all stages of a cell's life cycle. They're commonly used to treat a variety of cancers, particularly leukemia, because they're quite effective in killing cancer cells before they reproduce. Unfortunately, mesothelioma cancer hasn't responded well to anthracyclines in studies, so this class of chemo drug isn't normally used for mesothelioma.

- *Vinca alkaloids.* Vinca alkaloids target the process of cell division, called *mitosis*. These drugs interfere with the tiny structures that help move parts of DNA during cell division, thus preventing a cell from reproducing itself. Although few vinca alkaloids have proven to be effective in treating mesothelioma, researchers are investigating one of the newer agents, vinorelbine, which has shown promise in targeting mesothelioma cells. However, vinorelbine also presents some serious side-effect risks in many patients, so this agent hasn't yet moved into the standard treatment for mesothelioma.

> *The current standard chemotherapy for mesothelioma combines cisplatin and pemetrexed, which has proven to be the most effective treatment so far. The combination of agents attacks mesothelioma cells from two angles – pemetrexed interferes with cell metabolism, and cisplatin triggers a cell's "suicide" response. In addition, studies have indicated that most patients tolerate the toxic effects of cisplatin better when it's combined with pemetrexed.*

Researchers are investigating other types of anticancer agents that use other mechanisms to defeat cancer. Many of these agents are being tested in clinical trials (see the Experimental Treatments section later in this chapter for more information on what clinical trials are and how they work) and are not yet considered standard treatments for mesothelioma.

When Chemotherapy is Used

One of the most insidious traits of cancer cells is that they can detach themselves from the original site of the cancer, travel through your body and hide for months, even years, surviving without a blood supply until enough of them land in the same place to form a new tumor. Surgical techniques often can remove visibly diseased tissues and organs, but they can't guarantee that all of the cancer cells are gone. This is why many cancer patients – including mesothelioma patients – undergo both surgery and chemotherapy or radiation therapy (see the Radiation section later in this chapter). Chemo and radiation target cancer cells that surgery misses – what doctors call *occult disease.*

Chemo can be used before surgery to shrink a tumor, or after surgery to destroy cancer cells the surgery doesn't remove. When you undergo chemo before surgery, your doctor may use the term *neoadjuvant chemotherapy*. Chemo following surgery is called *adjuvant chemotherapy*. It's unclear whether chemo before surgery has any significant benefits for mesothelioma patients because this disease, unlike many other forms of cancer, tends to be *diffuse*, or spread out over a large area.

Most people think of chemo as a curative treatment; that is, chemo is often intended to kill all or most cancer cells in your body and send the cancer into *remission*. But chemo also may used as a palliative therapy – not intended to cure, but to manage the symptoms of your disease. (Given the side effects, however, some patients choose not to undergo chemo for palliative purposes.)

How Chemotherapy is Used

When your doctor discusses chemotherapy with you, he or she will likely use three terms to describe the treatment: *regimen*, *cycle*, and *course*. To the layperson, these terms seem interchangeable, but they have specific meanings when you're talking about chemo:

- A *chemotherapy regimen* describes the overall treatment plan. Your regimen will identify the chemo agent(s) the doctor will use; any secondary treatments, such as vitamin supplements to help your body better tolerate the effects of the chemo (for mesothelioma, folic acid and vitamin B12 are usually prescribed for this purpose); and the number and schedule of your treatments. The regimen is the complete roadmap of your chemo treatment.
- Chemotherapy regimens are considered either *first-line* or *second-line* therapies. First-line therapies are the standard treatments for a particular disease – for mesothelioma, first-line chemotherapy is the combination of cisplatin and pemetrexed (see "Types of chemo drugs" earlier in this chapter).

However, some patients don't respond well to first-line therapies; those patients typically receive second-line therapies. Unfortunately, there is no standard second-line chemotherapy for mesothelioma, but researchers are investigating several drugs that could become a second-line standard for this disease.

- A *chemotherapy cycle* is one leg of the journey on your chemo roadmap, consisting of one treatment and one resting period before the next treatment. The resting period gives your body time to recover from the side effects of the chemo. In addition, because chemo drugs target dividing cells and cells divide at different times, multiple cycles of chemo are more effective at killing off cancer cells than a single treatment would be.

  Delivering chemo on this treatment-and-rest cycle also helps the doctor determine how well your body tolerates the drugs being used and make adjustments to either the drugs or the dosage if needed.

- A *chemotherapy course* is the whole journey plotted out on your regimen. When you've completed all the treatment-and-rest cycles prescribed in the roadmap, you're done with your chemotherapy course. If the cancer reappears later, your doctor may recommend another course of chemotherapy.

Unless you're already hospitalized, you'll receive your chemo treatments on an outpatient basis. Sometimes chemo drugs are given in pill form or in a direct injection, but most commonly they're administered slowly through an IV drip. Your doctor may insert a port, usually in the chest, that will stay in throughout your chemotherapy course; when you come in for a treatment, the drugs will be administered through the port. After you've received the treatment, you'll return home (although you probably will want to have someone drive you to and from your treatment in case you experience nausea or other side effects from the drugs).

Researchers are looking into another delivery method called *isolated perfusion chemotherapy, or IPC*. Instead of circulating throughout your bloodstream, the chemo drugs are delivered into a particular area of the body, which tends to reduce side effects. This method also allows for the drugs to be heated, which improves their absorption by malignant cells and tissues. For mesothelioma patients, IPC is being studied in both the pleural surfaces (*intrapleural perfusion chemotherapy*) and in the abdomen (*intraperitoneal perfusion therapy*).

Radiation Therapy

Radiation therapy uses high-energy *ionizing* radiation to kill cancer cells. Ionizing radiation changes the structure of DNA in cells, thus inhibiting growth and division. Like chemotherapy, though, radiation therapy doesn't differentiate between healthy and cancerous cells, so the treatment damages normal cells as well. The side effects of radiation are similar to those for chemotherapy and include hair loss, digestive problems, and anemia.

Advances in radiation technology show promise in using this therapy to treat mesothelioma, although researchers are pushing for more studies to ensure that these new technologies are safe as well as effective. *External-beam radiation therapy* uses a machine to deliver targeted blasts of radiation to specific parts of the body. Combined with CT and MRI technology (see Chapter 3), radiation beams can be directed to target malignant tissues, thus minimizing the damage to healthy cells and tissues. This is important because your heart and lungs are highly sensitive to radiation, and the targeting ability affords some protection against unintended damage to these organs.

Most commonly, radiation therapy for mesothelioma involves targeted doses of radiation following surgery in locations where cancer cells are considered most likely to spread, such as around incision sites. At present, because of the risk of damaging critical organs and tissues, most doctors don't use radiation as a primary therapy for treating mesothelioma, but it has been proven useful and effective in combination with surgery.

New Therapies

Although chemotherapy, radiation and surgery remain the most common and conventional treatments for mesothelioma, researchers are investigating other treatments for this and other types of cancer. These experimental treatments include:

- *Gene therapy.* Gene therapy aims to target tumors without harming healthy cells by inserting a "suicide" gene directly into a tumor. This gene makes cancerous cells sensitive to drugs that normally aren't effective against cancer, and the drug affects only cancer cells. Gene therapy is in clinical trials to determine both its safety and effectiveness for large- scale use as a cancer treatment.

  > *Tip: Dr. Daniel Sterman at the NYU Langone Medical Center is a lead investigator using gene therapy in mesothelioma; see his entry in Appendix A (page 112).*

- *Photodynamic therapy.* Photodynamic therapy has shown promise in treating other forms of cancer and is now in the experimental stage for treating mesothelioma. The patient takes a drug called a ***photosensitizer*** that makes cells sensitive to light at specific wavelengths; the drug collects in cancerous cells but not in healthy cells. After the cancer cells are sensitized, a surgeon inserts fiber optic cables into the patient's body (typically through open-chest surgery) and beams the specific wavelength of light at the cancer cells. In response to the light, the drug produces a toxic oxygen molecule that kills the cancer cell.

  > *Tip: Dr. Joseph Friedberg is using photodynamic therapy at the University of Maryland School of Medicine; see his entry in Appendix A (page 111).*

- *Immunotherapy.* Immunotherapy (also called **biological therapy** or **BRM**, for **biological response modifiers**) aims to boost the body's immune system response to effectively isolate and kill cancerous cells. Like the other new therapies listed here, immunotherapy is being tested in clinical trials to determine its safety and effectiveness.

Clinical Trials

Clinical trials test the safety and effectiveness of drugs, medical devices, and surgical procedures in humans. These controlled tests typically have three or four phases. In Phase I trials, the focus is on safety, not effectiveness; researchers select a few dozen people (sometimes even fewer) to evaluate any side effects. If the drug, medical device or surgical procedure appears to be safe after Phase I, testing moves to Phase II, which involves several hundred people and lasts one to three years. Phase II trials measure both safety and effectiveness. Phase III trials are long-term studies – often eight to 10 years – to evaluate long-term safety and effectiveness; they typically involve between 1,000 and 3,000 patients and are implemented as part of the patients' regular medical care. Phase IV studies are carried out after the treatment has received federal approval and is available to anyone who needs it. The goal of Phase IV monitoring is to identify any potential problems with the treatment as well as other possible uses. For example, Phase IV monitoring led to the discovery that the antidepressant Wellbutrin is sometimes useful as a stop-smoking aid.

There are benefits and risks to participating in clinical trials. In all trials, patients are randomly selected to receive either the treatment being tested or a dummy treatment (called a *placebo*) that's harmless but also doesn't provide any benefit. In *single-blind trials*, the physician administering the treatment knows which patients are getting the real treatment and which are getting a placebo, but the patients don't know which treatment they're getting. In *double-blind trials* (which are considered more reliable), neither the patient nor the physician knows who's getting the real treatment and who's getting the placebo.

Clinicaltrials.gov has a searchable database of clinical trials around the world. You can use the database to get up-to-date information on the latest clinical trials for mesothelioma treatments, including trial locations, the kind of patients the trial's administrators are looking for, and what to expect if you apply for and are accepted for the trial. As always, be sure to talk with your doctor about your specific situation and the pros and cons of participating in such trials.

Finding a Doctor and Treatment Center

Although your primary care doctor may perform the initial evaluation and order tests, he or she should refer you to a mesothelioma specialist who will lead the medical team in confirming the diagnosis and formulating a treatment plan. Remember, mesothelioma is a rare form of cancer, and you'll get the best care from a doctor (and a facility) that specializes in this disease. Often, patients meet with two or more mesothelioma specialists to fully understand their options. Appendix A list mesothelioma treatment specialists, and recommended doctors and facilities are marked with an asterisk.

When you meet with a mesothelioma specialist (or any doctor, for that matter), it's a good idea to write down any questions you may have so you don't forget to ask while you're with the doctor. You also may want to have someone go with you to your appointments to help ensure you get the answers you need and understand any instructions or warning signs the doctor wants you to be aware of.

Here are some common questions mesothelioma patients want answered when they visit their doctor:

- What kind of mesothelioma do I have?
- What part of my body is affected?
- What stage is my mesothelioma?
- How do we know whether it has spread?
- What are my treatment options?
- What are the pros and cons of my treatment options?
- What are my chances of beating this?
- What should I expect during treatment?
- Is there anything else I can do to improve my chances or my quality of life?

You also may want to ask about the experience your doctor and treatment facility have with cases like yours. Don't be afraid to ask how many patients the doctor or hospital has treated or what their general experience has been with cases like yours.

> *It's important to see a mesothelioma specialist. These doctors will be most familiar with the disease and treatment options that can extend your life and improve the quality of your life.*

Your comfort level is just as important as their expertise. When you're considering doctors and treatment facilities, keep the following things in mind:

- Do you feel comfortable with the doctor and staff?
- Do the doctor and staff take the time to answer your questions and make sure you understand what they're telling you?
- Do the doctor and staff seem comfortable with answering your questions?
- Do you feel that the doctor and staff respect you as an individual?
- Does the doctor ask you how you feel about different treatment options?
- What will your care after surgery be like?

Several resources are available to help you locate appropriate doctors and treatment facilities. Some magazines, such as *U.S. News & World Report*, rank treatment centers according to their areas of expertise.

We've listed several doctors and treatment centers that specialize in mesothelioma in Appendix A of this book. You also can find doctors and treatment centers near you by visiting www.mesotheliomahelp.net.

Chapter 5

Living With Mesothelioma

There's no cure for mesothelioma, and the treatments discussed in Chapter 4 are aimed at either slowing the progress of the disease or relieving its symptoms. Coping with the diagnosis and the disease will take a toll on both your physical and emotional health, and your family and friends will feel its effects, too.

This chapter offers some tips for living with mesothelioma and keeping your quality of life as high as possible while you cope with the physical and emotional strains of the disease.

Taking Care of Your Physical Health

As with any other serious illness, mesothelioma (and other asbestos-related diseases) weakens your body and makes it difficult to do regular activities. In addition, the treatment you undergo has significant effects on your physical well-being.

In many cases, and especially in the early stages of the disease, diet, exercise, and relaxation techniques can help your body cope with the disease and the effects of your treatment—and thus make you feel better. The following sections explore these aspects of physical well-being in more detail.

Diet and Nutrition

Your appetite may be affected both by the disease and by your treatment. But getting enough food – and the right kind – is a key component in helping you feel better. Good nutrition helps your body fight infection and the side effects of your treatment, and eating well helps you maintain a healthy weight.

Different kinds of food provide different benefits for your physical health:

- *Protein* repairs tissues damaged by surgery, chemotherapy, and radiation. Protein also boosts your immune system and provides essential nutrients for cell and tissue growth. High-protein foods include beef, pork, chicken, and fish; cheese and other dairy products like milk, cottage cheese, and yogurt; nuts, seeds, and wheat germ; eggs; peanut butter; beans, peas, and tofu.
- *Fats and carbohydrates* provide energy to fuel your body. Although healthy individuals are generally advised to limit their fat and carb intake, cancer patients often need more of these kinds of foods to counter both their disease and the effects of their treatment. Fats are found in dairy products like butter, whole milk, buttermilk, and full-fat cheese, as well as some meats and products like peanut butter. High- carbohydrate foods include breads, pasta, and potatoes.
- *Vitamins and minerals* help your body digest food and absorb and use the nutrients in the food you eat. Depending on your overall health and diet, your doctor may recommend that you take a multivitamin or specific vitamin and mineral supplements to ensure your body gets the nutrition it needs.
- *Water* keeps your body hydrated, which in turn helps ensure that your body can use the nutrients you take in. Talk to your doctor about how much water you should drink each day.

Here are some good online resources about nutrition:

- American Cancer Society: Complete Guide to Nutrition for Cancer Survivors (www.cancer.org)
- Mayo Clinic: How to Get Nutrition When You Have No Appetite; Tips to Make Food Tastier; Alternative Cancer Treatment Options (www.mayoclinic.com/cancer and www.mayoclinic.com/cancer-treatment)

- Memorial Sloan-Kettering Cancer Center: Nutrition for Cancer Patients and other useful information (www.mskcc.org/cancer-care/survivorship)
- National Cancer Institute nutrition page (www.cancer.gov/cancertopics/pdq/supportivecare/nutrition)

You also may want to check out two books from the American Cancer Society: <u>American Cancer Society Complete Guide to Complementary and Alternative Therapies</u> and *American Cancer Society Complete Guide to Nutrition for Cancer Survivors*. Both are available from online booksellers.

> *Your doctor may prescribe a specific diet for you, and it's important to follow your doctor's instructions. After surgery, chemotherapy, or radiation treatments, for example, your doctor may want you to restrict or avoid certain foods while your body recovers from the treatment.*

Exercise and Relaxation

Several studies have shown that cancer patients who exercise feel better physically and emotionally. Exercise improves lung function, muscle strength, flexibility, and energy levels, and it releases chemicals in the brain called ***endorphins*** that help boost your mood and even can help you sleep better. Exercise also can help ease common side effects of cancer treatment, including nausea, fatigue, and diarrhea.

Yoga is often recommended for cancer patients because it combines low-impact physical movement with relaxation techniques. Many fitness centers offer regular yoga classes. You also may be able to practice yoga at home, either on your own or following a yoga DVD or video, as long as you have a quiet and comfortable place to do the breathing, stretching, and meditation exercises.

> *Your ability to do physical activity may be hampered by your disease, your overall health, and your treatment. Talk with your doctor about what kind of exercise is*

> *appropriate for your situation and how much exercise you should try to get every day or week. Also discuss whether you should participate in supervised exercise in a setting such as a rehab clinic or whether you can exercise on your own – via daily walks or swimming, for example.*

Pain Management

Dealing with pain from your disease or your treatment is one of the biggest challenges in maintaining and managing your quality of life. Your doctor may prescribe over-the-counter pain relievers such as aspirin, acetaminophen (the active ingredient in Tylenol), or ibuprofen. Prescription pain relievers typically are designed for short-term pain relief, such as immediately following surgery.

> *All pain relievers, including over-the-counter medications, can have negative effects on your kidneys, liver, and blood. Depending on what other medications you take and any other health issues you have, your doctor may limit your use of these drugs.*

Stretching and other forms of exercise may help with pain management (see the preceding section). Talk with your doctor before you start any exercise regimen, and be sure your doctor is aware of both the kind and intensity of any pain you experience.

Fatigue

Fatigue is one of the most common side effects of mesothelioma and its treatment. Although nearly everyone feels tired from time to time, fatigue from disease or aggressive treatment like chemotherapy interferes with daily activities and doesn't go away with rest.

Chemotherapy and radiation in particular can cause fatigue, because both these treatments affect the red blood cells in your body, leading to a condition called *anemia*.

When you have fewer red blood cells, your body doesn't get the oxygen it needs to function normally. Symptoms of anemia include feeling tired, weak, or dizzy; being short of breath; and inability to do, or lack of energy for, normal activities or tasks.

Your doctor can test your blood for anemia and may recommend dietary changes or nutritional supplements to combat or reverse its effects. In addition, you can adjust your lifestyle by:

- Planning several rest or short nap periods throughout your day.
- Saving your energy for the activities that are most important to you, and asking relatives and friends to take over or help you with routine tasks, such as household chores or errands.
- Taking part in "quiet" activities, such as reading, listening to music, or needlework.
- Joining a mesothelioma or cancer support group to share experiences and learn tips from others dealing with similar issues. Check out www.curemeso.org to find a group near you.

> *Mesothelioma patients often suffer from insomnia and other sleep disorders, which can be a result of either the disease or your treatment. Talk with your doctor if your sleep cycles or habits change significantly.*

You also may want to consider the following measures to promote more restful sleep:

- Ensure that your sleeping environment is quiet and dark, and that the air temperature is comfortable for you.
- Sleep in loose, soft clothing.
- Add or remove pillows to increase your comfort level.
- Go to the bathroom before you try to sleep.
- Avoid drinking anything with caffeine for at least two hours before bedtime.

- Eat a high-protein snack (if recommended or approved by your doctor) two hours before bed.
- Go to bed and get up at the same time every day.

Dealing with the Emotional Impact

Facing a serious illness can be emotionally devastating, especially when the disease is progressive and incurable. Patients often feel overwhelmed, frightened of what the future holds, and even depressed about their diagnosis. The patient's family and friends suffer emotionally, too, and may not know how to help the patient cope or how to express or deal with their own feelings.

> *Negative feelings are normal when you're diagnosed with mesothelioma or another serious illness, or when you learn that a relative or loved one has the disease. How you deal with your feelings can have a significant impact on your symptoms and your response to treatment, as well as your quality of life.*

The following sections discuss some common emotional issues that mesothelioma patients and their loved ones experience, along with some tips for coping with them.

Emotional Toll on the Patient

Anger, anxiety, fear, guilt, embarrassment, and depression all are common emotions after a mesothelioma diagnosis. These feelings can be especially strong if you had no major health issues or definite symptoms (see Chapter 3) before your diagnosis. When that's the case, learning that you have mesothelioma can feel like a kick in the gut, made even worse because of the shock.

Patients also may feel isolated, particularly because mesothelioma is a relatively rare disease. You may feel as though no one understands either your illness or your emotional pain. If you have to stop working because of the disease, you may feel a loss of identity, purpose, or meaning in your life.

Unfortunately, studies have shown that many *oncologists* (doctors who specialize in treating cancer patients) have a poor record of recognizing and correctly diagnosing the serious emotional turmoil their patients go through. That means it's even more critical that you talk with your doctor about any emotional or psychological symptoms you experience, because your mental health is just as important as your physical health in living with and treating your disease.

Signs to watch for include:

- *Depression.* Symptoms of depression include persistent sadness (daily or almost daily, and lasting for most of the day); overeating or loss of appetite, or significant weight gain or loss; lack of energy that isn't related to the effects of your treatment; loss of interest in things or activities you once enjoyed; feelings of guilt, hopelessness, or worthlessness; inability to sleep, or sleeping too much; thoughts of death or suicide.

- *Anxiety.* Anxiety can manifest itself in several ways, including difficulty thinking, making decisions, or solving basic problems; headaches, migraines, or other aches such as neck and shoulder pain; trembling, shaking, or restless movements; getting angry easily, especially over minor things.

> *Some of these symptoms are normal responses to your diagnosis and treatment. However, "normal" responses are generally temporary; you may feel incredibly anxious and depressed for a day or two, then return to your usual emotional state.*

If your symptoms of depression or anxiety persist, though, you should discuss options with your doctor or ask for a referral to a mental health specialist. Certain medications may help calm your symptoms, which in turn can make your treatment more effective and your day-to-day experience more enjoyable.

But because these medications may interact with others you may be taking, you should always consult your doctor first.

> *Exercise, proper nutrition, and relaxation techniques like yoga can help manage your emotional symptoms, too. See "Taking Care of Your Physical Health" earlier in this chapter.*

Many patients also find that joining a mesothelioma or cancer support group is helpful, particularly in fighting the sense of isolation that often accompanies the diagnosis. Knowing there are others who are facing similar challenges – and having a safe place to discuss your own experiences and feelings – can ease the emotional strain of coping with the realities of your disease and treatment.

Emotional Toll on Family and Friends

Relatives and friends are affected by a mesothelioma diagnosis just as profoundly (though in different ways) as the patient. Shock, grief, anger, and a sense of helplessness are common. Stepping into the role of a caregiver can be stressful, both physically and emotionally. Communication may become more difficult, as the patient may not wish to "burden" loved ones with his or her own feelings, and loved ones in turn may not feel free to share their own feelings or discuss important issues like end-of-life planning (see Chapter 8).

The following sections offer some insight into how your loved ones may react to your diagnosis and treatment, as well as suggestions for making the transition easier on you and your family and friends.

Your Relationship With Your Spouse

Your spouse is likely to be as frightened of your diagnosis as you are, and this fear may be compounded by anxiety over how to cope with your new needs and what the future holds. Your sex life also will be affected by the disease.

In some instances, the patient, the spouse, or both go into denial and refuse to discuss the illness or its implications. If this is the case, you may want to consider consulting a professional counselor who specializes in dealing with terminally ill patients and their families.

Ideally, your spouse should take part in discussions with your doctor about your treatment and your disease. Knowing the facts and what to expect can ease your spouse's anxiety and provide a stronger sense of partnership as you both face the challenges involved. In addition, being an active participant in these discussions can give your spouse a better sense of how he or she will be involved your care and what decisions the two of you will need to make (see Chapter 8 for information on end-of-life planning).

For the same reason, your spouse should be involved in discussions with your attorney if you file a legal claim (see chapters 6 and 7) so he or she knows what to expect from the process.

Children

Even adult children can have a hard time coping with a parent's illness. Losing a parent is never easy, and your children may not feel confident in their ability to "take over" the role of supporter during your illness. They may feel guilty about having limited time or resources to offer, especially if they have families and jobs of their own, and they may find the stress of additional responsibilities overwhelming.

Your children also may not know how to communicate their feelings of anger, fear, or guilt, or how to let you express your own feelings to them. It's important that both you and your children are able to acknowledge your feelings without either of you feeling guilty for doing so.

Discussing ways in which your children can help you and your spouse – such as performing household chores or running errands, or even planning regular visits – can help ease stress for everyone, because then your children know what you want and need from them, and you and your spouse know what kind of help and support you can expect from your children.

Other Loved Ones

Other people in your family and circle of friends also will be affected by your diagnosis. Parents, siblings, and in-laws may be able to help with emotional support and certain tasks; or, if you've been accustomed to helping them, you may have to ask other family members to take on those responsibilities or find other alternatives for their care and support.

Friends may find it difficult to discuss your disease or treatment, and they may not know exactly how to show their support. You can ease the strain by asking for specific assistance when they say, "If there's anything I can do…" You may ask friends to stay with you while your spouse goes out to run errands or for a social engagement that you don't feel up to attending, for example. Or you may ask friends to provide a social outing for your spouse as a break from his or her new responsibilities.

> *If you're honest about what you want and need from your family and friends, your relationships will be stronger and your quality of life will be better. Let people know when you need company, and be honest when you just don't feel up to it. Offers of help are positive measures of your loved ones' feelings for you, so give yourself permission to accept these offers in the spirit in which they're given.*

Considering Hospice Care

Hospice programs provide so-called "comfort care" to patients whose illnesses have stopped responding to treatment, or to patients who choose not to pursue aggressive treatment. Nearly every community in the country has a hospice program; your doctor or local hospital can refer you to your local hospice group.

You can receive hospice care in your home or at a residential facility or nursing home. Medicare and other insurance plans often cover most hospice costs.

The goal of hospice care is to make the patient as comfortable as possible during the final months of life. In addition to pain management and other medical treatments, hospice programs typically offer spiritual support to the patient and loved ones.

Hospice workers also can discuss end-of-life considerations with you and your family, such as advance directives, do not resuscitate orders, and funeral planning (see Chapter 8). Family members also have access to counseling and bereavement services when a patient dies while in hospice care.

> *Choosing hospice care is a valid option and often relieves both physical and emotional stress for patients and their families. Because mesothelioma is resistant to treatment and because the treatment options for this disease have serious side effects, some patients elect to focus on the quality of their lives rather than on attempting to extend their lives.*

Your doctor can refer you to hospice programs near you. Just as you should feel comfortable with your doctor and attorney, you should choose hospice services you feel comfortable with and that are experienced in helping patients with your disease. Most hospice programs are open to patients who are expected to live six months or less.

Chapter 6

Exploring Your Legal Rights and Options

Many illnesses are *idiopathic*, meaning of unknown cause; no specific substance is responsible for causing the disease. Mesothelioma is different because its only known cause is exposure to asbestos.

For decades, asbestos companies knew of its dangers, yet they failed to take the simple steps that would have protected tens of thousands of workers and consumers – and their families – from these dangers. Most asbestos companies failed to put warnings on their products or use substitute materials. In fact, many companies went to great pains to keep the known dangers of asbestos secret from both their workers and the public. They put profits before safety.

This bad behavior is why most people with mesothelioma and other asbestos-related diseases file lawsuits – to hold asbestos companies responsible and to get compensation for their injuries.

In this chapter, we explain your rights and options as a victim of asbestos exposure. First, we explain the time limits in your state for filing legal claims for asbestos-related disease. Then we provide advice for finding the right attorney for you and your family. Finally, we provide an overview of the various kinds of financial help that may be available to you so you know which options to discuss with your attorney.

Filing a Timely Claim

To protect and assert your rights as a mesothelioma patient (or victim of another asbestos-related disease), you have to act quickly after you've received your diagnosis.

Every state has placed a time limit, called a *statute of limitation*, on mesothelioma claims. The clock starts ticking as soon as you receive your initial diagnosis, and if you don't file your claim within the specified time frame, you lose many of your rights to compensation. In addition, because many people with mesothelioma live less than a year after diagnosis, it's important to act quickly.

Here are the statutes of limitations for each of the 50 states and the District of Columbia:

Statute of Limitations Chart

1 year	Kentucky, Louisiana, Tennessee
2 years	Alabama, Alaska, Arizona, Arkansas, California, Colorado, Connecticut, Delaware, Georgia, Hawaii, Idaho, Illinois, Indiana, Iowa, Kansas, Minnesota, Nevada, New Jersey, Ohio, Oklahoma, Oregon, Pennsylvania, Texas, Virginia, West Virginia
3 years	District of Columbia, Maryland, Massachusetts, Michigan, Mississippi, Montana, New Hampshire, New Mexico, New York, North Carolina, Rhode Island, South Carolina, South Dakota, Vermont, Washington, Wisconsin
4 years	Florida, Nebraska, Utah, Wyoming
5 years	Missouri
6 years	Maine, North Dakota

Choosing an Attorney

The laws and options surrounding mesothelioma and asbestsos-related disease claims are varied and complex, and you'll want the help of a qualified and experienced mesothelioma attorney to help you decide which options make the most sense for you and your family.

Find an experienced mesothelioma lawyer who has tried mesothelioma cases in court (gone to verdict) as well as negotiated out-of-court settlements, and is respected nationally as a mesothelioma attorney. It's also important to hire an attorney who will actually work on your case – not one who will refer your case to another law firm. Many lawyers advertise for mesothelioma cases, but they don't actually work those cases; instead, they refer you to another lawyer. You should avoid this situation.

> *To protect your legal rights, you should contact an attorney as soon as possible after you've been diagnosed with mesothelioma or any asbestos-related disease. It's best to choose an attorney or law firm with significant experience in asbestos-related cases, but you also want an attorney you feel comfortable with.*

Here are some things to look for when shopping for an attorney:

- *Experience.* The attorney should give you an overview of his or her experience and success rate in mesothelioma cases.

- *Attention.* Your attorney should listen to the specifics of your case, understand and address any concerns you have, and explain your options – and the pros and cons of each option – in language you can understand. Your attorney also should make recommendations based on your specific case.

- *Fairness.* Attorneys who work with mesothelioma patients typically accept cases on a contingency basis, which means they don't get paid unless they win your case or negotiate an acceptable settlement. Contingency fees are usually a percentage of a settlement or jury award – generally between 33.3 and 40 percent of the total money received. Make sure you understand what percentage your attorney will take and whether there will be any expenses in addition to that percentage, such as postage, travel, or other expenses, and get the fee agreement in writing. Expenses should be taken out of the total settlement, not your share of the proceeds.

- *Responsiveness.* Does the attorney (or someone from the firm) return your calls promptly? Do they answer your questions fully and courteously?

- *Comfort.* You should feel comfortable talking and working with your attorney, just as you should feel comfortable dealing with your doctor. If you don't feel comfortable, don't hesitate to check out other attorneys.

Your first meeting with an attorney, called an *initial consultation*, should be free, and the attorney should offer to come to your home. During that first meeting, here are some questions you may want to ask:

- What is your experience (or the firm's experience) successfully trying mesothelioma cases and lawsuits?
- How many cases have you handled?
- Will you handle the case, or will you refer it to another law firm?
- If you accept my case, will I be working with you or with someone else in your office? Who else will be on my legal team?
- What are my legal options, and which options do you recommend?
- What are the chances of success in my case?
- If you accept my case, how long will it take to receive my compensation?
- Will my case be part of a class-action lawsuit, or will it be an individual suit?
- Will I have to go to trial to resolve my case, or will it be settled out of court?
- If I'm too sick to work with you, will you work with a member of my family on my behalf?
- How will you protect my privacy within the firm and in dealing with potential defendants?

> *Be wary of law firms that send investigators or other non-lawyers to your initial meeting. You are hiring a lawyer, not a professional investigator or marketer – and you should be meeting with a lawyer, not someone who travels around signing up cases.*

> *Relatives may be able to file suit on behalf of someone who has died from mesothelioma or another asbestos-related illness, as long as the claim is filed within the time frame dictated by law. Contact an attorney to find out what your options are.*

Belluck & Fox has a national reputation as asbestos and mesothelioma attorneys. We have recovered more than $500 million for our clients with mesothelioma and asbestos-related cancers, and Belluck & Fox has been named one of the top law firms in the United States.

Checking Out Financial Assistance Options

A mesothelioma diagnosis often includes a hefty financial burden. If you don't already have health insurance, you likely won't qualify for a new health insurance plan. Even if you have health insurance, your out-of-pocket expenses for doctor's appointments, tests, treatments, and prescriptions may go up significantly – and some treatments may not be covered at all. You'll also likely spend more on transportation to and from various appointments and may have to spend more on meals and other travel-related expenses, depending on how far you live from your doctor and/or treatment center. You also may want to participate in experimental treatments, which typically are not covered by insurance.

Most mesothelioma patients have several avenues available to them to help out with the costs associated with their illness. The following sections describe some of these options. Be sure to discuss these with your attorney; in some cases, filing certain claims may limit your rights to other forms of compensation. It's important to have your mesothelioma lawyer handle all your compensation benefit claims to make sure you're fully protected.

Individual Lawsuits

If you decide to file a lawsuit, your attorney will seek both compensatory and punitive damages. *Compensatory damages* cover your economic losses – such as medical expenses, lost income, and any additional costs related to your illness, and your non-economic damages, such as compensation for pain and suffering. *Punitive damages* are designed to punish the company (or companies) for their negligence or other bad behavior in exposing you to the risks of asbestos. Lawsuits also can recover damages for your spouse's loss of companionship.

Your attorney will look at several factors in your case, including:

- *Your work and life history.* An experienced attorney will take a detailed history to identify every way you may have been exposed to asbestos at work and at home – even from dust and fibers carried into your home by a household member who worked with or was exposed to asbestos. Because so many products (ranging from car brake pads to floor tiles) contained asbestos, it's not uncommon for people to be unaware or unable to remember how they were exposed. (See Chapter 1 for information on *direct* and *indirect exposure*.) Experienced mesothelioma attorneys have a vast store of knowledge and resources to identify how and where you may have been exposed to asbestos – and who is responsible for that exposure.

- Your eligibility to file a claim, including whether your claim is timely.

  > *If you're a smoker and have mesothelioma or another asbestos-related illness, you are still eligible to file a claim. Smoking and asbestos exposure both can cause lung cancer, and these two factors combined increase your risk for developing lung cancer.* **However, smoking does not cause mesothelioma, asbestosis, or other asbestos-related diseases.** *If you've been diagnosed with one of these diseases, the cause is asbestos exposure and your smoking habits have nothing to do with your illness.*

- *Your rights under various bankruptcy trust funds.* Your attorney will determine your eligibility for payment from mesothelioma trust funds established under bankruptcy proceedings.

- *Existing documents and new evidence pertaining to your circumstances.* Your attorney should have an extensive library of documents and testimony from other asbestos cases that can be used in developing your case. In addition, your attorney may interview you and other witnesses (such as co-workers, medical experts, and so on) to help build your case.

- *Who should be sued.* Even if you don't remember where or when you may have been exposed to asbestos, your attorney can help you determine these details by examining your work history and other facts. Generally, the defendants in an asbestos exposure case include the manufacturer(s) of asbestos-containing products; contractors that installed and/or repaired asbestos-containing products and equipment; suppliers of materials to the work site; and property owners who allowed asbestos to be used on their property.

- *What is a fair level of compensation for your suffering?* An experienced mesothelioma attorney will be able to give you a rough idea of what your claim should be worth, based on the circumstances of your case and the outcome of similar cases. However, it's important to remember that each case is different. While most attorneys won't accept your case unless they believe it has a very good chance of being successful, no attorney should make any promises about the amount of compensation you'll receive. Instead, as your case progresses, your attorney will evaluate any offers based on what he or she feels is fair and reasonable compensation for you. (See Chapter 7 for more on how your case will proceed.)

Mesothelioma Trust Funds

Many companies that manufactured asbestos products have filed for bankruptcy protection to avoid making huge payouts to injured workers and their families. In many cases, bankruptcy judges have ordered the companies to establish trust funds specifically for victims of asbestos-related illnesses. (The nearby sidebar lists some asbestos companies that have declared bankruptcy or are no longer in business as of this writing, but have active trust funds for asbestos claims.) These trust funds pay at a very reduced rate, and the proceeds from these funds aren't enough to fully compensate you.

Your attorney can help you determine whether you have a legitimate claim against one of the mesothelioma trust funds. These claims must be coordinated with your lawsuit, because they can affect other attempts to win compensation for your illness.

Asbestos Companies with Active Bankruptcy Trust Funds

As of 2010, 54 asbestos companies had filed for bankruptcy and established trust funds to deal with claims of asbestos-related diseases. Other companies are awaiting court approval for their bankruptcy trust funds; your attorney will have up-to-date information.

The following page contains a partial list of asbestos companies with active bankruptcy trust funds.

Active Bankruptcy Trust Funds

AC&S (ARMSTRONG)	Keene Corp.
API, Inc.	Lake Asbestos of Quebec, Ltd.
Armstrong World Industries	National Gypsum (GOLD BOND)
Babcock and Wilcox Co.	Owens Corning Corp. (KAYLO)
Carey Canada, Inc.	Owens Corning Fibreboard
Celotex Corp.	Plibrico Co.
Combustion Engineering	Porter-Hayden Co.
Congoleum Corp.	Raymark Corp./Raytech (RAYBESTOS)
Eagle-Picher Industries	Stone and Webster Engineering
GAF (DELCO)	T. H. Agriculture and Nutrition, LLC
General Motors	Unarco
Harbison-Walker	USG (United States Gypsum) Corp.
H. K. Porter Co.	Western MacArthur/Western Asbestos
Johns-Manville Corp. (TRANSITE)	W.R. Grace

Class Action Lawsuits

Class action lawsuits involve a large group of people who suffer similar injuries or wrongdoing at the hands of the same defendant(s). Class action lawsuits aren't used in mesothelioma and asbestos cases. Class action suits most often are settled out of court and therefore often appeal to people who don't want to go to trial. However, because of the large number of *claimants* (those suing for damages), settlements in these cases are typically based on the broadest interests of the class. Individual circumstances that may warrant a larger settlement amount aren't considered in class action cases.

The lack of consideration for individual circumstances is the main reason that the U.S. Supreme Court has ruled that class action lawsuits aren't appropriate for asbestos cases. People who are exposed to asbestos have widely differing circumstances, including different exposure levels, different ages, different diseases, and different medical treatment. Such variety makes it virtually impossible to craft a class action settlement that would be fair to every member of the class.

Other Kinds of Assistance

Depending on your circumstances, you may be eligible to receive other kinds of assistance to help you with the financial impact of your illness. You should discuss these options with your attorney, who can tell you more about the process of applying for these forms of assistance and the impact such applications may have on your case.

- *Worker's compensation.* If you worked for an asbestos company, you may also have the right to file a claim. In most states, you cannot sue your employer, but you can file a worker's compensation claim. The laws governing worker's compensation claims vary from state to state and can be extremely confusing. Your attorney can explain your options and the pros and cons if you want to file a claim against your (current or former) employer.

- *Veterans' benefits.* Many members of the military were exposed to asbestos during their service. You may be eligible to file a claim with the Department of Veterans Affairs.

- *Social Security disability benefits.* If your asbestos related illness has forced you to quit working before you reach retirement age, you may be eligible for Social Security disability benefits. Again, filing for these benefits can be complex and confusing, so talk with your attorney about the filing process and what you can expect.

- *Medicare/Medicaid coverage.* If you're over age 65, you should qualify for Medicare coverage. However, Medicare itself doesn't cover all medical expenses. If you're transitioning from an employer health insurance plan to Medicare, your out-of-pocket expenses could increase significantly, depending on what kind of supplemental Medicare insurance you purchase. Medicaid is a state-federal health insurance program that covers low-income individuals and families. Be sure to check with your attorney or ask for a referral to a Medicaid expert to stay up-to-date on changes in coverage, eligibility, and other factors.

- *Long-term disability insurance.* If you don't already have a long-term disability insurance policy before you're diagnosed with mesothelioma, you probably won't qualify for a new policy. However, if you're already covered before your diagnosis, this policy should begin paying benefits (usually a percentage of your former salary) after you've been disabled for six months. Check with your employer's human resources department or with the insurance carrier to find out when your benefit kicks in, how much you'll receive, whether your payments from the policy are taxable, and the policy's time limits. Most policies only pay out for two or three years because they assume that, if you're permanently disabled, you'll apply for and receive Social Security disability benefits.

- *Community assistance programs.* Many communities have organizations that help arrange such things as transportation to and from doctor visits, home-delivered meals, help with household chores or errands, and financial assistance with out-of-pocket expenses. Your local chapter of the American Cancer Society should be able to provide referrals to this kind of help in your community.

Chapter 7

How the Claims Process Works

Filing a lawsuit can be confusing, and this is especially true in asbestos-related cases because such lawsuits usually involve more than one defendant and often involve filings outside of court, such as claims to bankruptcy trusts.

This chapter walks you through the basic steps of filing a mesothelioma lawsuit, from initial consultation to court verdict or out-of-court settlement. Laws and regulations on the process vary from state to state, so be sure to ask your attorney to explain the requirements that pertain to your case.

Stages of a Lawsuit

Although every case has unique circumstances and facts, the process of consulting with an attorney and filing a lawsuit follows the same basic pattern: initial contact, preparation, filing the lawsuit, answer phase, deposition, and then settlement or trial. If a case goes to trial, there may also be an appeals process.

> *Because of the aggressive nature of mesothelioma and lung cancer, most state allow for expedited schedules for mesothelioma cases. Your attorney should do everything he or she can to fast-track your case and resolve your claims within six to 12 months. Cases are usually filed within 30 days of the initial consultation, and depositions typically are completed within 30 to 60 days of filing. The attorney handling your case will attempt to make your case move even faster if your health warrants quicker action.*

The following sections explain these stages in more detail.

Initial Contact

Your first contact with an attorney usually involves a brief telephone conversation to get some basic facts about your case and determine whether you should pursue a legal claim. If the attorney believes you have a valid case, the next step is scheduling a face-to-face meeting to discuss your case, your legal options, and the process of filing and prosecuting a lawsuit.

This in-person meeting should be with a lawyer – not a paralegal or investigator. The lawyer should offer to come to your home for the in-person meeting so that you don't have to travel if you don't want to.

> *If you choose to have Belluck & Fox represent you, the firm will schedule your in-person meeting within 24 hours whenever possible. We will have our attorney visit you in your home. During this meeting, the attorney will go over your work, life, and medical history and ask you to sign release forms (also called "authorizations") that allow the firm to get copies of your medical and employment records.*

You'll also sign a ***retainer agreement*** that spells out when and how – and how much – the lawyer will be paid if your lawsuit is successful. You should hire a lawyer who works on a ***contingency basis***, meaning they don't get paid unless they win an award for you, either in a trial or an out-of-court settlement. If you do win an award, the law firm's fee will be deducted from your award.

Preparation

After the initial meeting, your attorney will research your case to determine who should be named as defendants (see Chapter 6 for information on who typically gets sued in asbestos-related cases) and in which court your claim should be filed. Because laws in every state are different, one of the most important decisions is where to file your claim; typically, your claim will be filed in the state where you live or where you were exposed to asbestos. Your attorney will explain these options to you. An experienced mesothelioma attorney will already have records from most asbestos companies and information on major job sites and Navy ships. They'll use this information to help research your case.

Filing the Complaint

When the research is completed, your attorney will file your complaint in the appropriate court. The companies named as defendants will be served with copies of the complaint. The complaint typically will assert that the defendants are responsible for manufacturing, selling, and/or installing defective products and equipment, that they caused your asbestos exposure, and that they failed to warn you of the dangers of that exposure.

Answer Phase

Defendants usually have 30 days to respond to lawsuits filed against them. In asbestos-related cases, defendants will send your lawyer a response to the allegations in the lawsuit. After the court receives the defendants' responses, the court will hold a hearing and scheduling conference for the case, allotting a certain amount of time – usually between six and 12 months – for both sides to prepare their case (see the following section) and schedule a trial date.

Discovery Phase

The *discovery phase* of your case gives both your attorney and the defendants time to interview witnesses, obtain needed documents, and conduct other research pertaining to your lawsuit. Both your attorney and the defendants will hire medical and other experts to review your case; these experts may be called to testify if your case goes to trial.

Deposition

As the plaintiff, you'll be required to give a *deposition*, or sworn testimony given outside of a courtroom. Depositions can take place at your attorney's office, a court reporter's office, or at a convenient location for all parties, such as a hotel conference room. If necessary, your attorney may arrange for your deposition to take place at your home. Your attorney should choose a place that's convenient to do.

Prior to your deposition, your attorney will meet with you to go over the questions that will be asked and prepare you for the deposition. The people present at your deposition will include you, your attorney, the court reporter (who takes a transcript of everything said during the deposition), and attorneys representing the defendants. Your deposition also may be recorded via audio or video.

Your attorney will ensure that the questions you're asked are fair and reasonable and relate to your lawsuit. On occasion, he or she may object to a question and instruct you not to answer. Depending on the complexity of your case and the number of defendants, your deposition may take a couple of hours or may last longer.

The defendants' attorneys will be looking to find out how you were exposed to asbestos. You should be prepared for them to ask questions about your medical and work history.

After your deposition, your attorney and the defendants' attorneys will receive copies of the transcript. Evidence you give in your deposition may be used in court if your case goes to trial. Your attorney also may do a second videotaped deposition for use at trial, in which your attorney asks questions as if you were in the courtroom. This videotape will be played during your trial if you're unable to participate.

> *Except for your deposition, your attorney will perform most, if not all, of the work required during the discovery phase.*

> *The release forms you sign at your first meeting permit your attorney to get copies of your medical and work records, so you won't even have to collect those documents.*

Trial / Settlement Phase

When your claim is first filed, both your attorney and the court will assume that there will be a trial in your case. However, most mesothelioma and other asbestos-related cases are settled out of court before a trial begins. There are several reasons why your case may settle:

- The defendant(s) may see that the evidence in your favor is overwhelming, making it unlikely that they would succeed at trial.
- The defendant(s) may wish to avoid the time and expense of a trial.

Settlement offers can come at any time after your claim is filed, even up to – or during – a trial. Your attorney will evaluate any settlement offers and discuss them with you.

> *You don't have to accept any offer if you feel it's unfair. An experienced mesothelioma attorney can advise you on whether a given offer is reasonable for your circumstances, but the decision on whether to accept a settlement or proceed to trial is ultimately yours to make.*

Many people prefer to settle over going to trial, because trial outcomes are unpredictable. In addition, if you receive a large award from a jury, one or more of the defendants in your case is likely to appeal the award, which obviously lengthens the process (see the following section). Settlement offers often include provisions that require you to keep the terms of the settlement private and usually state that the defendant does not admit to any wrongdoing. For some people, the lack of accountability in a settlement offer is a deal-breaker; they want the companies responsible for their asbestos exposure and illness to be held publicly accountable for their actions, so they prefer to go to trial. Only you can decide whether a settlement offer is acceptable to you.

If you agree to a settlement, the defendant(s) will send your attorney a check for the full settlement amount. Your attorney will then send you a check for your portion; you also should receive a statement of deducted expenses with your check. You shouldn't have to wait until the end of your case to receive settlement money.

If your case involves multiple defendants, you may receive a settlement offer from some defendants but not from others. If that happens and you accept the settlement offers, those defendants will be dismissed from your complaint and you will continue to trial with the remaining defendants.

If your case goes to trial, your attorney will present testimony and evidence in support of your claim, including the testimony of expert witnesses. You may have to be present in court and testify at trial.

The length of a trial depends largely on the complexity of your case. Some trials take only a week, plus the time for the jury to deliberate; others may last several weeks or longer. Your attorney can give you an idea of how long a trial might last in your case.

If you win at trial, the jury will award you a sum of money. This award may be reduced by your previous settlements and other benefits you received, such as worker's compensation.

Appeals

Defendants who lose at trial usually have between 30 and 180 days (six months) to file an appeal. An appeal delays any payment to you, but the defendant usually must post a ***bond***, or security for the amount awarded at trial, until the appeal is resolved.

Appeals most often adjust the amount of the award given at trial; in some cases, an appeals court may order a new trial.

If the defendant loses the appeal, the trial award stands. If the defendant wins the appeal, you'll receive the new award determined by the appeals court (or no payments at all if the appeals court reduces the award to zero or orders a new trial).

> *If your attorney works on a contingency basis and you lose on appeal, you do not have to pay your attorney out of your own pocket. Your attorney only gets paid from money you're awarded in a trial (and possible appeal) or a settlement.*

Other Claims

Your attorney will file the other claims mentioned in Chapter 6 at some point during this process. Ask your attorney about the timing of these other claims, such as worker's compensation and bankruptcy trust claims.

Chapter 8
Other Legal Considerations

Although treatments for mesothelioma have improved over the years, it remains an incurable and progressive disease. Survival times after diagnosis depend largely on how early your mesothelioma is diagnosed, what type of mesothelioma you have (see Chapter 1), and how it responds to treatment, as well as your general health and genetic predisposition to fighting off disease.

Eventually, though, your symptoms and overall health will worsen, and you may reach a point where you're unable to make health care decisions for yourself. Planning ahead for this time can do much to ease the stress you and your family will feel as you deal with your illness.

This chapter covers basic end-of-life issues that every family affected by mesothelioma must face. Making sure your affairs are in order helps ensure that your wishes are carried out and gives your loved ones a guide if they have to make decisions on your behalf.

Advance Health Care Directives

Advance health care directives, often called "living wills," provide written instructions for your health care in the event you can't make decisions yourself or are unable to communicate what you want. The rules and regulations for advance health care directives vary from state to state; your doctor or attorney can tell you what's required in your state.

Advance directives also provide instructions for life-saving and life-sustaining treatments. Without an advance directive of some sort, emergency responders will do everything they can to keep you alive and stabilize your condition; for example, if you have a heart attack, they will attempt to get your heart beating again in regular rhythm unless you've left instructions for them not to attempt to resuscitate you (called a DNR order, for Do Not Resuscitate).

> *You can refuse any medical treatment you don't want, and you can put limits on the types of treatment you do want. For example, if you have to be put on a ventilator or other life-sustaining treatment (such as a feeding tube), you can include a time limit after which your doctor and loved ones must discuss your chances of recovery and decide whether to continue or stop the treatment.*

The most effective advance directives are fashioned after careful consideration and discussion with your loved ones. It's not an easy thing to contemplate or talk about, and sometimes it's less uncomfortable to have this discussion on a "what if" basis. For many people, the toughest question is deciding when the quality of life is poor enough to stop treatment.

Here are some "what if" questions to help you get started:

- What if you can't breathe on your own? Do you want to be put on a ventilator? How long are you willing to be kept on a ventilator?
- What if you're unable to eat? Do you want to have a feeding tube? How long do you want to survive on a feeding tube?
- What if your chances of recovery are 50-50?
- What if your chances of recovery are good, but you're likely to need round-the-clock medical care?

You also may want to discuss these scenarios with your doctor or health care team (including home health aides and social workers, if you have them). If they know what your wishes are, they can help you and your loved ones navigate tough decisions when the time comes. In addition, your doctor can give you an idea of the kinds of complications and late-stage situations that you and your loved ones may have to face.

You should put your wishes in writing; many medical centers and law firms have standard forms you can fill out. File your advance directive with your will and other important papers and make sure your loved ones know where to find it should they need it.

This document should include:

- Instructions for your treatment in an emergency (such as a Do Not Resuscitate order)
- Instructions regarding life-sustaining treatments such as ventilators and feeding tubes, as well as time limits or other limitations you want to establish
- Instructions for evaluating the outcome of your treatment and determining whether you would find those outcomes acceptable
- A health care proxy – someone who's authorized to make decisions about your medical treatment if you're unable to make or communicate your wishes yourself.

Wills

In addition to an advance health care directive, you should have a will that describes how your money, property, and personal effects are to be distributed after your death. If you die intestate – that is, without a will – whatever cash and possessions you leave behind will be distributed according to the laws of the state in which you live. These laws may or may not coincide with what you want.

Drafting a will is relatively inexpensive, and it can save your loved ones a lot of headaches. Your attorney can either draw one up for you or refer you to another lawyer who specializes in wills and estate planning.

Some things don't need to be included in your will. If you have life insurance, for example, the proceeds from that policy will be paid to the person or people you named as beneficiaries when you purchased it. You can list your estate as the beneficiary if you want the money from the policy to be pooled with your other assets. The same is true for certain retirement accounts, such as 401(k)s, and may be true for other financial holdings like CDs or money-market accounts. If you have or are eligible to receive a pension from your employer, check with your human resources department to find out what you need to do to ensure your spouse or children can claim pension funds after your death.

Other Important Papers

Your loved ones should know where to find:

Insurance policies, including contact information (if not an agent's name and phone number, then the phone number for the life insurance company)

- Deeds, titles, and other ownership papers for real estate, autos, and other titled property
- Rental agreements for safe deposit boxes, post office boxes, storage units, etc.
- Bank account information
- Retirement account information, including pensions, IRAs, 401(k)s, and so on
- Any documentation related to your work history, asbestos exposure, and lawsuit

> *If you die before your case is resolved, either by settlement or jury verdict (see Chapter 7), your claim can proceed. Your estate will receive any award and the proceeds will be divided among your survivors. In addition, your spouse or children may be able to file a wrongful death lawsuit; your attorney, who is already familiar with your case, can advise your family of their rights and options.*

Glossary

Term	*Definition*
asbestosis	Scarring of the lung tissue as a result of inhaling the microscopic fibers in asbestos dust.
adjuvant chemotherapy	Chemotherapy after surgery, designed to attack cancer cells the surgery missed.
advance health care directive	Written instructions for your health care in the event you can't make decisions yourself or are unable to communicate what you want.
alveoli	Air sacs at the ends of bronchioles that transfer oxygen into your blood stream and absorb carbon dioxide.
anthracyclines	Chemotherapy drugs that damage a cell's DNA and thus interfere with all stages of a cell's life cycle; generally ineffective against mesothelioma.
antifolates	Chemotherapy drugs that inhibit cell growth and division by interfering with DNA replication.
apoptosis	A process in which a cell is pre-programmed to "commit suicide" if its growth gets out of control or it is damaged.
benign	Non-cancerous
biological response modifiers (BRM)	See entry: immunotherapy
biological therapy	See entry: immunotherapy

Term	Definition
biphasic mesothelioma	Mesothelioma composed of a combination of epithelial and sarcomatoid cancer cells.
bronchi	The large airways that branch off from your trachea into your lungs; each large airway is called a bronchus.
bronchioles	Smaller airways that reach deep into your lungs.
chemotherapy	The use of chemicals to destroy cancerous cells.
chemotherapy course	The complete number of chemotherapy cycles.
chemotherapy cycle	One treatment and one resting period before the next chemotherapy treatment.
chemotherapy regimen	The overall chemotherapy treatment plan.
cilia	Tiny hairs that line your bronchial tubes and sweep dust and other particles out of your airways.
cisplatin	The oldest of the chemo platinum agents; still considered the standard (in combination with pemetrexed) for mesothelioma chemotherapy.
claimant	The person or organization claiming damages in a lawsuit.
class action	A type of lawsuit in which there are a few identified plaintiffs representing the interests of many others who are in similar situations.
clinical trials	Experiments on humans that test drugs, surgeries, and medical devices for safety and effectiveness.

Term	Definition
compensatory damages	Recovery of actual economic losses, such as lost income, medical expenses and other actual costs or losses.
contingency basis	A fee arrangement in which your attorney only gets paid if he or she wins a monetary award for you.
contrast material	A special dye that provides sharper images by highlighting or outlining certain parts of your body.
CT scan (computed tomography)	Imaging technique that uses x-rays and computers to draw more detailed pictures of your internal organs.
curative	Intended to cure.
debulking pleurectomy	A surgical procedure to remove as much cancer from the pleura as possible to ease pressure on the lungs; often combined with pleurodesis
decortication	A procedure in which the layer of fibrous tissue surrounding the lung is removed.
defendant	The person or organization being sued.
deposition	Sworn testimony given outside of a courtroom.
diaphragm	The muscle that separates your chest cavity from your abdominal cavity.
diffuse	Spread out over a large area.
discovery	The phase in a lawsuit in which attorneys for both sides collect evidence and interview witnesses.
double-blind trials	Clinical trials in which neither the patients nor the doctors administering the trial know who receives the actual treatment and who receives a placebo.
dyspnea	Shortness of breath.

Term	_Definition_
epiglottis	A small flap of tissue that prevents food and liquid from going into your lungs when you swallow.
epithelial	Relating to the surface layers of membranes.
excisional biopsy	A procedure in which an entire abnormal mass is removed for testing.
external-beam radiation therapy	A technique that uses a machine to deliver targeted blasts of radiation to specific parts of the body.
extrapleural pneumonectomy	A surgery similar to pleurectomy/decortication, but the surgeon also removes the affected lung; usually done when the mesothelioma has spread beyond the pleura and has begun infiltrating the lung, or when asbestos-related lung cancer is present in addition to mesothelioma
first-line therapy	Standard treatment for a disease.
gene therapy	An experimental technique that aims to kill cancer cells by inserting a "suicide" gene.
health care proxy	Someone who's authorized to make decisions about your medical treatment if you're unable to make or communicate your wishes yourself.
histology	A cell's type characteristics.
immunostains	Special dyes that make abnormal cells stand out under a microscope.
immunotherapy	Immunotherapy aims to boost the body's immune system response to effectively isolate and kill cancerous cells; also called biological therapy or BRM (biological response modifiers).

Term	Definition
incisional biopsy	A procedure in which a portion of an abnormal mass is removed for testing.
initial consultation	First meeting, usually with a professional such as a doctor or lawyer.
intestate	Lack of a will detailing how your assets are to be divided after your death.
intraperitoneal perfusion therapy	An IPC technique being studied for mesothelioma, in which chemotherapy drugs are delivered directly to the lining of the abdomen.
intrapleural perfusion chemotherapy	An IPC technique being studied for mesothelioma, in which chemotherapy drugs are delivered directly into the lining of the lung.
ionizing radiation	A specific kind of radiation that changes the structure of DNA in cells, thus inhibiting growth and division.
isolated perfusion chemotherapy (IPC)	A technique in which chemo drugs are delivered into a particular area of the body rather than circulated throughout the bloodstream.
laparoscopy	A procedure that uses a tiny scope to examine the pleura and other areas of the abdominal cavity.
laparotomy	A procedure in which samples of the abdominal pleura are taken to test for mesothelioma.
latency period	The period between exposure to a disease-causing agent and the onset of symptoms of the disease.
macroscopically complete resection	Removal of all visibly diseased or damaged organs and/or tissues.
malignant	Cancerous

Term	_Definition_
mediastinoscopy	A procedure in which the scope is inserted under the sternum to view lymph nodes and take samples.
mesothelium	A thin membrane that protects your internal organs and allows them to move freely without damage-causing friction.
Mitosis	The process of cell division.
MRI (magnetic resonance imaging)	Imaging technique that uses a magnetic field and radio waves to scan your body.
multimodal treatment	The combination of two or more kinds of treatment, such as surgery and chemotherapy.
neoadjuvant chemotherapy	Chemotherapy before surgery, usually used to shrink a tumor.
occult disease	Disease at a cellular level, invisible to the naked eye.
oncologist	Doctor who specializes in treating cancer patients.
palliative	Treatment or actions intended to relieve symptoms, but with no curative intent or ability.
paracentesis	A procedure used to drain excess fluid in the abdomen and collect samples for testing and diagnosis.
pathologist	A doctor who specializes in identifying and studying the nature, causes, and progression of disease.
pemetrexed	An antifolate drug commonly used in mesothelioma chemo treatments.
pericardium	Mesothelium around the heart.

Term	Definition
peritoneum	The mesothelium that protects your abdominal cavity (stomach, intestines, and other organs).
PET (positron emission tomography)	Imaging technique that measures functional activity in your body.
PET-CT scan	A machine that combines CT and PET technology and can provide your doctor with a better overall picture of your physical health.
photodynamic therapy	An experimental technique that makes cancer cells vulnerable to light at specific wavelengths.
placebo	A dummy treatment that does no harm but doesn't affect a disease or illness.
plaintiff	The person or organization who files a lawsuit against a defendant; also called claimant.
platinum agents	Chemotherapy drugs that attack a cell's DNA and disrupt its structure, thus triggering the cell's pre-programmed "suicide" response (apoptosis).
pleura	Mesothelium surrounding your lungs.
pleural effusion	A build-up of fluid in the pleura.
pleural plaques	Localized areas of scar tissue that forms around asbestos fibers.
pleurectomy/decortication	Surgery involving removing the pleura and peeling away the fibrous layer around the lung.
pleurodesis	Surgical procedure in which the pleura lining the lungs and the chest wall and diaphragm are fused to prevent fluid build-up and pleural effusions.

Term	*Definition*
port	An implanted medical device that allows easy access for IVs.
punitive damages	Money ordered paid as punishment for bad behavior.
radiation therapy	A technique that uses high-energy ionizing radiation to kill cancer cells.
retainer agreement	A contract that spells out how and how much your attorney gets paid.
sarcomatoid	Involving cells from bone and muscle.
secondary exposure	Indirect exposure to a contaminant, such as asbestos fibers carried home on a worker's clothing.
second-line therapy	Standard treatment alternatives when patients don't respond to first-line therapies.
single-blind trials	Clinical trials in which the doctor administering the trial knows which patients are receiving the actual treatment and which are receiving a placebo.
spirometry	Lung function test.
statute of limitations	Time limit in which certain actions, such as filing a lawsuit, must be taken.
sternum	The breastbone.
thoracentesis	A procedure in which samples are taken for testing and excess fluid is drained to help make the patient more comfortable.
thoracic cavity	The area of the torso from the neck to the diaphragm, containing the heart and lungs.
thoracotomy	Surgery that involves cutting through the chest wall to access the thoracic cavity and internal organs.

Term	Definition
thorascopy	A procedure that uses a tiny scope to examine the pleura and other areas of the chest cavity.
thorax	The upper part of the torso.
trachea	The windpipe.
video-assisted thoracic surgery (VATS)	A less invasive form of thoracic surgery, in which a smaller incision is made and the surgeon uses a tiny camera to view the heart and lungs.
vinca alkaloids	Chemotherapy drugs that target the process of cell division (mitosis) by interfering with the tiny structures that help move parts of DNA during cell division.
wrongful death	Death resulting from negligence or willful wrongdoing.

Appendix A
Mesothelioma Specialists

Because mesothelioma is a relatively rare disease, it's important to seek out a specialist and treatment center with experience in treating this form of cancer. Use this list to find a doctor and treatment center near you. If your state isn't listed, ask your primary doctor for a referral to a cancer specialist or treatment center.

Physicians and treatment centers marked with an asterisk (*) are recommended.

Mesothelioma Specialists & Treatment Centers

Arizona

Dr. Linda L. Garland

University of Arizona Cancer Center - North Campus
3838 N. Campbell Ave.
Tucson, AZ 85719

(520) 626-3434

Dr. Helen J. Ross

Mayo Clinic
13400 E. Shea Blvd.
Scottsdale, AZ 85259

(800) 446-2279

California

Dr. Joel Baumgartner

Moores Cancer Center
3855 Health Sciences Dr
La Jolla, CA 92093

(800) 926-8273

California

* Dr. Robert B. Cameron   UCLA Medical Center
10780 Santa Monica
Boulevard, Suite 100
Los Angeles, CA 90025

(310) 470-8980

Dr. Mark R. Cullen   Stanford University School of Medicine
1265 Welch Rd
MSOB X-338, MC 5414
Stanford, CA 94305

(650) 721-6209

Dr. Michael Y. Chang   Kaiser Foundation Hospital - Los Angele
4760 Sunset Blvd #3
Los Angeles, CA 90027

(323) 783-7510

* Dr. David M. Jablons   UCSF Medical Center at Mount Zion
Helen Diller Family Comprehensive Cancer Center
1600 Divisadero Street, Fourth Floor
San Francisco, CA 94143

(415) 885-3882

Dr. Thierry Marie Jahan   UCSF Medical Center at Mount Zion
Helen Diller Family Comprehensive Cancer Center
1600 Divisadero Street, Fourth Floor
San Francisco, CA 94143

(415) 885-3882

Dr. Mark W. Lischner   Pulmonary Medicine Associates
5 Medical Plaza Drive, Suite 190
Roseville, CA 95661

(916) 786-7498

Colorado

* Dr. Paul A. Bunn

University of Colorado Denver
School of Medicine
Division of Medical Oncology
Anschutz Medical Campus
13001 E. 17th Place
Aurora, CO 80045

(303) 724-4499

Connecticut

Dr. Constantinos A. Constantinou

94 Union Street
Rockville, CT 06066

(860) 870-1300

Dr. Frank Detterbeck

Smilow Cancer Hospital
at Yale-New Haven
Thoracic Oncology Program
35 Park Street, Ste 4th Floor
New Haven, CT 06511

(203) 200-5864

Dr. Scott Gettinger

Yale Cancer Center

Yale New Haven Hospital
South Frontage Road and Park St.,
4th Floor
Multispecialty Care Center
New Haven, CT 06510

(203) 200-5864

Dr. Michael R. Grey

The Hospital of Central Connecticut
100 Grand Street
New Britain, CT 06050

(860) 224-5661

Dr. James V. Lettera

Bridgeport Hospital
267 Grant St
Bridgeport, CT 06610

(203) 922-7870

Connecticut

Dr. Thomas James Lynch
Smilow Cancer Hospital
at Yale-New Haven
South Frontage Road and Park St.,
4th Floor
Multispecialty Care Center
New Haven, CT 06510

(203) 200-5864

Dr. Michael Teiger
New England Integrative Health Associates
345 North Main Street, Suite 101
West Hartford, CT 06117

(860) 278-3812

Florida

* Dr. Scott J. Antonia
Moffitt Cancer Center
12902 Magnolia Drive
Tampa, FL 33612

(813) 745-8412

Dr. Clay M. Burnett
Cardiovascular Surgeons, P.A.
217 Hillcrest Street
Orlando, FL 21801

(401) 425-1566

* Dr. Lary Robinson
Moffitt Cancer Center
12902 Magnolia Drive
Tampa, FL 33612

(813) 745-8412

Georgia

Dr. Peter W. Barrett

Piedmont Heart Institute
95 Collier Road Northwest, Suite 5015
Atlanta, Georgia 30309

(404) 605-5699

Dr. David M. Berkowitz

Winship Cancer Institute of
Emory University
1365 Clifton Road NE
Atlanta, GA 30322

(404) 778-3755

Dr. Daniel L. Miller

Cancer Treatment Centers of America
Southeastern Regional Medical Center
600 Celebrate Life Parkway
Newnan, GA 30265

(800) 931-9299

Hawaii

Dr. Michele Carbone

University of Hawaii
701 Ilalo Street
Honolulu, HI 96813

(808) 586-3013

Illinois

Dr. Philip D. Bonomi

Rush University Cancer Center
Section of Medical Oncology
1725 W. Harrison Street, Suite 1010
Chicago, IL 60612

(312) 942-5904

Dr. Hedy Lee Kindler

University of Chicago Cancer Research
Center - Center for Advanced Medicine
5758 S. Maryland Avenue
Chicago, IL 60637

(855) 702-8222

Illinois

Dr. Michael J. Liptay — Rush University Cancer Center
Rush Professional Office Building
1725 W. Harrison Street, Suite 774
Chicago, IL 60612

(312) 738-3732

Dr. Wickii Thambiah Vigneswaran — University of Chicago Medical Center - Center for Advanced Medicine
5758 S. Maryland Avenue
Chicago, IL 60637

(773) 702-3351

Kentucky

Dr. Terry E. Justice — Tri-State Regional Cancer Center
706 23rd St
Ashland, KY 41101

(606)-329-0060

Dr. Jeffrey P. Lopez — Tri-State Regional Cancer Center
706 23rd St
Ashland, KY 41101

(606)-329-0060

Dr. Timothy W. Mullett — University of Kentucky College of Medicine
740 S. Limestone Street, Suite A301
Lexington, KY 40536-0284

(859) 323-6494

Maine

Dr. Seth D. Blank — MaineGeneral Medical Center
35 Medical Center Parkway, 1st Flr.
Augusta, Maine 04330

(207) 861-6550

Maryland

Dr. Richard H. Alexander — University of Maryland Medical Center
22 S. Greene Street
Baltimore, MD 21201

(410) 328-6897

* Dr. Joseph S. Friedberg — University of Maryland School of Medicine
22 S. Greene Street
Executive Office, Suite N9E17
Baltimore, MD 21201

(410) 328-6366

* Dr. Stephen C. Yang — Sidney Kimmel Comprehensive Cancer Center at Johns Hopkins
600 N. Wolfe Street Blalock 240
Baltimore, MD 21287

(410) 614-3891

Massachusetts

Dr. Raphael Bueno — Brigham and Women's Hospital
75 Francis Street
Boston, MA 02115

(617) 732-6824

Dr. Neal Chuang — 299 Carew Street, Suite 410
Springfield, MA 01104

(413) 748-9628

Dr. Marcelo DaSilva — Brigham and Women's Hospital
75 Francis Street
Boston, MA 02115

(617) 732-6824

Dr. Tammy Gleeson — Southcoast Physicians Group Thoracic Surgery
208 Mill Road Pod F
Fairhaven, MA 02719

(508) 973-2204

Massachusetts

* Dr. Pasi A. Janne — Dana-Farber Cancer Institute
450 Brookline Avenue
Boston, MA 02215

(617) 632-6875

Dr. Abraham Lebenthal — Brigham and Women's Hospital
75 Francis Street
Boston, MA 02115

(617) 732-6824

Dr. Laki Rousou — 299 Carew Street, Suite 410
Springfield, MA 01104

(413) 748-9628

Dr. Scott Swanson — Brigham and Women's Hospital
75 Francis Street
Boston, MA 02115

(617) 732-6824

Michigan

Dr. Frank Baciewicz, Jr. — Barbara Ann Karmanos Cancer Institute
4100 John R Street
Detroit, MI 48201

(800) 527-6266

Dr. Peter W. Barrett — Borgess Health
1535 Gull Road, Suite 130
Kalamazoo, MI 49048

(269) 345-1161

Dr. Richard Berri — **St. John Hospital and Medical Center
22101 Moross Rd
Detroit, MI 48236**

(313) 647-3252

Michigan

Dr. Shirish M. Gadgeel — University of Michigan
Comprehensive Cancer Center
7217 Cancer Center
1500 E Medical Drive, SPC 5948
Ann Arbor, MI 48109-5948

(734) 647-6883

* Dr. Michael Harbut — St. John Providence
29275 West 10 Mie Road
Farmington Hills, MI 48336

(248) 849-3107

Dr. Lourens J. Willekes II — Metro Hospital Wyoming MI
4500 Cascade Road SE, Suite 210
Grand Rapids, MI 49546

(616) 259-7341

Nebraska

* Dr. Brian Loggie — CHI Health Clinic - Surgical Oncology
(Bergan)
7710 Mercy Road, Suite 2000
Omaha, NE 68131

(402) 717-0090

Nevada

* Dr. Nicholas Vogelzang — Comprehensive Cancer Centers of
Nevada
3730 S. Eastern Avenue
Las Vegas, NV 89169

(702) 952-3400

New Hampshire

Dr. David J. Finley   Norris Cotton Cancer Center
                             Dartmouth-Hitchcock Medical Center
                             One Medical Center Drive
                             Lebanon, NH 03756

                             (603) 650-8537

Joseph D. Phillips   Norris Cotton Cancer Center
                             Dartmouth-Hitchcock Medical Center
                             One Medical Center Drive
                             Lebanon, NH 03756

                             (603) 650-8537

New Jersey

* Dr. Jean-Phillippe Bocage   Thoracic Group, PA
  &   35 Clyde Road, Suite 104
  Dr. Robert J. Caccavale   Somerset, NJ 08873

                               (732) 247-3002

Dr. Bruno N. Cole   JFK Medical Center - New Jersey
                               65 James St
                               Edison, NJ 08820

Dr. Bruce G. Haffty   The Cancer Institute of New Jersey
                               195 Little Albany Street
                               New Brunswick, NJ 08903

                               (732) 235-8515

Dr. Frederic Seinfeld   St. Francis Medical Center
                               601 Hamilton Ave, RM 109
                               Trenton, NJ 08629

                               (609) 599-5307

Dr. Loki Skylizard   Monmouth Medical Center
                               300 2nd Ave
                               Long Branch, NJ 07740

                               (417) 820-3960

New Jersey

* Dr. Federico Steiner & Dr. Mark D. Widmann

North Jersey Thoracic Surgical Associates
100 Madison Avenue
Morristown, NJ 07960

(973) 644-4844

New York

Dr. Manjit Bains

Memorial Sloan-Kettering Cancer Center
1275 York Avenue
New York, NY 10021

(212) 639-7450

Dr. Mark J. Crye

Upstate University Hospital
4835, 750 East Adams Street
Syracuse, NY 13210

(315) 464-6257

* Dr. Raja M. Flores

Mount Sinai Medical Center
1470 Madison Avenue
New York, NY 10029

(212) 241-9466

Dr. Nicholas Karis

Genesee Valley Cardiothoracic, P.C.
1415 Portland Avenue, Suite 240
Rochester, New York 14621

(585) 922-3260

Dr. Leslie J. Kohman

Upstate University Hospital – SUNY
750 East Adams Street, 4835
Syracuse, NY 13210

(315) 464-3510

Daniel Labow

Mount Sinai
1000 10th Ave
New York, NY 10019

(212) 241-2891

New York

Dr. Bernard Park — Memorial Sloan-Kettering Cancer Center
1275 York Avenue
New York, NY 10021

(646) 888-3346

* Dr. Harvey Pass — NYU Langone Medical Center
160 East 34th Street, 8th Fl.
New York, NY 10016

(212) 731-5414

Dr. Roman Perez-Soler — **Montefiore Medical Center**
MMC Medical Park at Eastchester
1695 Eastchester Road
Bronx, NY 10461

(718) 405-8505

Dr. Christian G. Peyre — **University of Rochester Medical Center**
601 Elmwood Avenue
Box SURG
Rochester, NY 14642

(585) 275-1509

Dr. Dennis J. Rassias — **Albany Thoracic and Esophageal Surgery, PLLC**
319 S. Manning Blvd, Suite 206
Albany, NY 12208

(518) 525-8501

* Dr. Kenneth Rosenzweig — Mount Sinai Medical Center
1184 Fifth Ave., 1st Floor
New York, NY 10029

(212) 241-5095

New York

* Dr. Valerie Rusch

Memorial Sloan-Kettering Cancer Center
1275 York Avenue
New York, NY 10021

(212) 639-5873

Dr. Daniel Sterman

NYU Langone Medical Center
160 East 34th Street, 8th Fl.
New York, NY 10016

(212) 731-6162

Dr. Jason Wallen

Upstate University Hospital – SUNY
750 East Adams Street, 8141
Syracuse, NY 13210

(315) 464-6255

North Carolina

Dr. David H. Harpole, Jr.

Duke University Medical Center
2301 Erwin Road
Durham, NC 27710

(919) 668-8413

Ohio

Dr. Claire Verschraegen

Ohio State University –
Comprehensive Cancer Center
The James Cancer Hospital and Solove Research Institute
460 West 10th Avenue,
Columbus, Ohio 43210

(614) 293-0463

Oklahoma

Dr. Daniel Nader — CTCA Southwestern Regional Medical Center
10109 E. 79th Street (81st Street & Highway 169)
Tulsa, OK 74133

(918) 286-5000

Pennsylvania

Dr. Steven M. Albelda — University of Pennsylvania Cancer Center - Penn Lung Center
3615 Civic Center Boulevard
Philadelphia, PA 19104

(215) 615-5864

Dr. Evan W. Alley — Penn Mesothelioma and Pleural Program
Penn Medicine University City
3737 Market Street, 4th Floor
Philadelphia, PA 19104

(215) 662-9801

Dr. Charles T. Bakhos — Temple University Hospital
3401 N. Broad Street
Ambulatory Care Center,
5th Floor (Zone D)
Philadelphia, PA 19140

(215) 707-9115

Dr. David Bartlett — Mesothelioma Specialty Care Center of UPMC Cancer Centers
Hillman Cancer Center
5115 Centre Avenue
Pittsburgh, PA 15232

(412) 692-2852

Pennsylvania

Dr. Neil A. Christie
Mesothelioma Specialty Care Center of UPMC Cancer Centers
Hillman Cancer Center
5115 Centre Avenue
Pittsburgh, PA 15232

(412) 623-2025

Dr. Cherie P. Erkmen
Temple University Hospital
3401 N. Broad Street
Ambulatory Care Center,
5th Floor (Zone D)
Philadelphia, PA 19140

(215) 707-9115

Dr. Colleen Gaughan
Penn Medicine
Lancaster General Hospital
555 North Duke Street
Lancaster, PA 17602

(717) 544-9400

Dr. Larry Kaiser
Temple University School of Medicine
3500 N. Broad Street, 11th Floor
Philadelphia, PA 19140

(215) 707-7000

Dr. Rodney J. Landreneau
Landreneau Thoracic Surgical Associates
600 Medical Arts Building
Kittanning, PA 16201

(724) 548-3813

Dr. James D. Luketich
Mesothelioma Specialty Care Center of UPMC Cancer Centers
200 Lothrop Street, Suite C-800
Pittsburgh, PA 15213

(412) 647-7555

Pennsylvania

	Dr. James Pingpank	Mesothelioma Specialty Care Center of UPMC Cancer Centers Hillman Cancer Center 5115 Centre Avenue Pittsburgh, PA 15232 (412) 692-2852
*	Dr. Michael F. Reed	Penn State Hershey Thoracic Surgery 500 University Drive Cancer Institute T1400 Hershey, PA 17033 (717) 531-6585
	Dr. Matthew J. Schuchert	University of Pittsburgh Medical Center 200 Lothrop St Pittsburgh, PA 15213 (412) 623-1128
	Dr. Sunil Singhal	Hospital of the University of Pennsylvania Division of Thoracic Surgery 3400 Spruce Street, 6th Floor, White Bldg Philadelphia, PA 19104
*	Dr. Jennifer Toth	Penn State Hershey Pulmonary Medicine 500 University Drive Hershey, PA 17033 (717) 531-6525

Tennessee

Dr. Eric S. Lambright	The Vanderbilt Clinic
1301 Medical Center Drive, Suite 1710
Nashville, TN 37232

(615) 322-0064

Dr. Spence McCachren	Thompson Oncology Group
1915 White Ave
Knoxville, TN 37916

(865) 331-1720

Texas

Dr. Kemp Kernstine	UT Southwestern Simmons Cancer Center
University Hospital Thoracic Surgery Clinic
2201 Inwood Road
Dallas, Texas 75390

(214) 645-4673

* Dr. David Rice	University of Texas
M.D. Anderson Cancer Center
1515 Holcombe Boulevard, Unit 1489
Houston, TX 77030

(713) 792-2121

* Dr. W. Roy Smythe	The Texas A&M University System Health Science Center
2401 South 31st Street
Temple, TX 76508

(254) 724-2111

* Dr. David Sugarbaker	Baylor College of Medicine
Lung Institute (Clinic)
6620 Main Street, Suite 1325
Houston, Texas 77030

(713) 798-6376

Texas
* Dr. Anne Tsao

University of Texas
M.D. Anderson Cancer Center
1515 Holcombe Boulevard, Unit 0432
Houston, TX 77030

(713) 792-6363

Utah
Dr. Amit N. Patel

Huntsman Cancer Institute -
University of Utah
2000 Circle of Hope
Salt Lake City, UT 84112

(801) 585-0303

Vermont
Dr. Bruce J. Leavitt

Fletcher Allen Health Care
111 Colchester Ave
Burlington, VT 05401

(802) 847-4044

Dr. Michael C. Norotsky

Fletcher Allen Health Care
111 Colchester Ave
Burlington, VT 05401

(802) 847-4152

Virginia
Dr. Joan H. Schiller

Inova Schar Cancer Institute
3225 Gallows Rd
Fairfax, VA 22031

(571) 472-0250

Washington

* Dr. Eric Vallieres

Swedish Cancer Institute at
Swedish Medical Center
1101 Madison Street, Suite 850
Seattle, WA 98104

(206) 215-6800

Washington, D.C.

* Dr. Paul H. Sugarbaker

Washington Cancer Institute
106 Irving Street NW, Suite 3900
Washington, DC 20010

(202) 877-3908

Appendix B

Personal Medical Journal

Use these pages to keep track of your medications, symptoms, treatments, and contact information for your health care team. You can also use the "Notes" section to write down questions for your next doctor visit.

My Primary Physician

Name: _____

Address: _____

City: _____

State: _____

Zip: _____

Phone: _____

Email: _____

My Specialist Physician

Name: _____
Specialty: _____
Address: _____
City: _____
State: _____
Zip: _____
Phone: _____
Email: _____

My Specialist Physician

Name: _____
Specialty: _____
Address: _____
City: _____
State: _____
Zip: _____
Phone: _____
Email: _____

My Specialist Physician

Name: _____
Specialty: _____
Address: _____
City: _____
State: _____
Zip: _____
Phone: _____
Email: _____

My Specialist Physician

Name: _____
Specialty: _____
Address: _____
City: _____
State: _____
Zip: _____
Phone: _____
Email: _____

My Pharmacy

Pharmacy: _____
Pharmacist: _____
Address: _____
City: _____
State: _____
Zip: _____
Phone: _____
Prescriptions: _____
_____
_____
_____

My Pharmacy

Pharmacy: _____
Pharmacist: _____
Address: _____
City: _____
State: _____
Zip: _____
Phone: _____
Prescriptions: _____
_____
_____

My Medications

Drug: _____

Dosage: _____ Frequency: _____

Refill Date: _____

To Treat: _____

Drug: _____

Dosage: _____ Frequency: _____

Refill Date: _____

To Treat: _____

Drug: _____

Dosage: _____ Frequency: _____

Refill Date: _____

To Treat: _____

Drug: _____

Dosage: _____ Frequency: _____

Refill Date: _____

To Treat: _____

My Medications

Drug: _____

Dosage: _____ Frequency: _____

Refill Date: _____

To Treat: _____

Drug: _____

Dosage: _____ Frequency: _____

Refill Date: _____

To Treat: _____

Drug: _____

Dosage: _____ Frequency: _____

Refill Date: _____

To Treat: _____

Drug: _____

Dosage: _____ Frequency: _____

Refill Date: _____

To Treat: _____

My Medications

Drug: _____

Dosage: _____ Frequency: _____

Refill Date: _____

To Treat: _____

Drug: _____

Dosage: _____ Frequency: _____

Refill Date: _____

To Treat: _____

Drug: _____

Dosage: _____ Frequency: _____

Refill Date: _____

To Treat: _____

Drug: _____

Dosage: _____ Frequency: _____

Refill Date: _____

To Treat: _____

My Medications

Drug: _____

Dosage: _____ Frequency: _____

Refill Date: _____

To Treat: _____

Drug: _____

Dosage: _____ Frequency: _____

Refill Date: _____

To Treat: _____

Drug: _____

Dosage: _____ Frequency: _____

Refill Date: _____

To Treat: _____

Drug: _____

Dosage: _____ Frequency: _____

Refill Date: _____

To Treat: _____

Medical Allergies / Side Effects

Hospital / Treatment Facility

Hospital: _____
Contact: _____
Address: _____
City: _____
State: _____
Zip: _____
Phone: _____
Email: _____

Hospital / Treatment Facility

Hospital: _____
Contact: _____
Address: _____
City: _____
State: _____
Zip: _____
Phone: _____
Email: _____

Hospital / Treatment Facility

Hospital: _____
Contact: _____
Address: _____
City: _____
State: _____
Zip: _____
Phone: _____
Email: _____

Hospital / Treatment Facility

Hospital: _____
Contact: _____
Address: _____
City: _____
State: _____
Zip: _____
Phone: _____
Email: _____

Hospitalization Record(s)

Dates: _____

Hospital: _____

Physician: _____

Reason /
Diagnosis: _____

Prognosis /
Treatment: _____

Dates: _____

Hospital: _____

Physician: _____

Reason /
Diagnosis: _____

Prognosis /
Treatment: _____

Dates: _____

Hospital: _____

Physician: _____

Reason /
Diagnosis: _____

Prognosis /
Treatment: _____

Hospitalization Record(s)

Dates: _____

Hospital: _____

Physician: _____

Reason /
Diagnosis: _____
_____

Prognosis /
Treatment: _____
_____

Dates: _____

Hospital: _____

Physician: _____

Reason /
Diagnosis: _____
_____

Prognosis /
Treatment: _____
_____

Dates: _____

Hospital: _____

Physician: _____

Reason /
Diagnosis: _____
_____

Prognosis /
Treatment: _____
_____

Hospitalization Record(s)

Dates: _____

Hospital: _____

Physician: _____

Reason /
Diagnosis: _____
_____

Prognosis /
Treatment: _____
_____

Dates: _____

Hospital: _____

Physician: _____

Reason /
Diagnosis: _____
_____

Prognosis /
Treatment: _____
_____

Dates: _____

Hospital: _____

Physician: _____

Reason /
Diagnosis: _____
_____

Prognosis /
Treatment: _____
_____

My Health History

Date: _____ Time: _____ Duration: _____

Symptoms / Side Effects: _____

Location: _____

Action: _____

Date: _____ Time: _____ Duration: _____

Symptoms / Side Effects: _____

Location: _____

Action: _____

Date: _____ Time: _____ Duration: _____

Symptoms / Side Effects: _____

Location: _____

Action: _____

Date: _____ Time: _____ Duration: _____

Symptoms / Side Effects: _____

Location: _____

Action: _____

My Health History

Date: _____ Time: _____ Duration: _____

Symptoms / Side Effects: _____

Location: _____

Action: _____

Date: _____ Time: _____ Duration: _____

Symptoms / Side Effects: _____

Location: _____

Action: _____

Date: _____ Time: _____ Duration: _____

Symptoms / Side Effects: _____

Location: _____

Action: _____

Date: _____ Time: _____ Duration: _____

Symptoms / Side Effects: _____

Location: _____

Action: _____

My Health History

Date: _____ Time: _____ Duration: _____

Symptoms /
Side Effects: _____
_____

Location: _____

Action: _____

Date: _____ Time: _____ Duration: _____

Symptoms /
Side Effects: _____
_____

Location: _____

Action: _____

Date: _____ Time: _____ Duration: _____

Symptoms /
Side Effects: _____
_____

Location: _____

Action: _____

Date: _____ Time: _____ Duration: _____

Symptoms /
Side Effects: _____
_____

Location: _____

Action: _____

My Health History

Date: _____ Time: _____ Duration: _____

Symptoms / Side Effects: _____
_____

Location: _____

Action: _____

Date: _____ Time: _____ Duration: _____

Symptoms / Side Effects: _____
_____

Location: _____

Action: _____

Date: _____ Time: _____ Duration: _____

Symptoms / Side Effects: _____
_____

Location: _____

Action: _____

Date: _____ Time: _____ Duration: _____

Symptoms / Side Effects: _____
_____

Location: _____

Action: _____

My Health History

Date: _____ Time: _____ Duration: _____

Symptoms / Side Effects: _____

Location: _____

Action: _____

Date: _____ Time: _____ Duration: _____

Symptoms / Side Effects: _____

Location: _____

Action: _____

Date: _____ Time: _____ Duration: _____

Symptoms / Side Effects: _____

Location: _____

Action: _____

Date: _____ Time: _____ Duration: _____

Symptoms / Side Effects: _____

Location: _____

Action: _____

Notes

Appendix C

Mesothelioma Treatment Record

Use these pages to keep track of surgeries, chemotherapy, and radiation therapy treatments, as well as any side effects you may experience.

My Biopsies

Date: _____   Biopsy Type: _____

Reason: _____

Complications: _____

_____

Side Effects: _____

_____

Date: _____   Biopsy Type: _____

Reason: _____

Complications: _____

_____

Side Effects: _____

_____

Date: _____   Biopsy Type: _____

Reason: _____

Complications: _____

_____

Side Effects: _____

_____

My Surgeries

Date: _____ Surgery Type: _____
Reason: _____
Complications /
Side Effects: _____

Date: _____ Surgery Type: _____
Reason: _____
Complications /
Side Effects: _____

Date: _____ Surgery Type: _____
Reason: _____
Complications /
Side Effects: _____

Date: _____ Surgery Type: _____
Reason: _____
Complications /
Side Effects: _____

My Chemotherapy

Date: _____   Cycle: _____

Medications: _____

Complications /
Side Effects: _____

Next Appt: _____

Date: _____   Cycle: _____

Medications: _____

Complications /
Side Effects: _____

Next Appt: _____

Date: _____   Cycle: _____

Medications: _____

Complications /
Side Effects: _____

Next Appt: _____

Date: _____   Cycle: _____

Medications: _____

Complications /
Side Effects: _____

Next Appt: _____

My Chemotherapy (continued)

Date: _____ Cycle: _____

Medications: _____

Complications /
Side Effects: _____

Next Appt: _____

Date: _____ Cycle: _____

Medications: _____

Complications /
Side Effects: _____

Next Appt: _____

Date: _____ Cycle: _____

Medications: _____

Complications /
Side Effects: _____

Next Appt: _____

Date: _____ Cycle: _____

Medications: _____

Complications /
Side Effects: _____

Next Appt: _____

My Chemotherapy (continued)

Date: _____ Cycle: _____

Medications: _____

Complications /
Side Effects: _____

Next Appt: _____

Date: _____ Cycle: _____

Medications: _____

Complications /
Side Effects: _____

Next Appt: _____

Date: _____ Cycle: _____

Medications: _____

Complications /
Side Effects: _____

Next Appt: _____

Date: _____ Cycle: _____

Medications: _____

Complications /
Side Effects: _____

Next Appt: _____

My Chemotherapy (continued)

Date: _____ Cycle: _____

Medications: _____

Complications /
Side Effects: _____

Next Appt: _____

Date: _____ Cycle: _____

Medications: _____

Complications /
Side Effects: _____

Next Appt: _____

Date: _____ Cycle: _____

Medications: _____

Complications /
Side Effects: _____

Next Appt: _____

Date: _____ Cycle: _____

Medications: _____

Complications /
Side Effects: _____

Next Appt: _____

My Radiation Treatments

Date: _____ Session: _____

Treatment: _____

Complications /
Side Effects: _____

Next Appt: _____

Date: _____ Session: _____

Treatment: _____

Complications /
Side Effects: _____

Next Appt: _____

Date: _____ Session: _____

Treatment: _____

Complications /
Side Effects: _____

Next Appt: _____

Date: _____ Session: _____

Treatment: _____

Complications /
Side Effects: _____

Next Appt: _____

My Radiation Treatments (continued)

Date: _____ Session: _____

Treatment: _____

Complications /
Side Effects: _____

Next Appt: _____

Date: _____ Session: _____

Treatment: _____

Complications /
Side Effects: _____

Next Appt: _____

Date: _____ Session: _____

Treatment: _____

Complications /
Side Effects: _____

Next Appt: _____

Date: _____ Session: _____

Treatment: _____

Complications /
Side Effects: _____

Next Appt: _____

My Radiation Treatments (continued)

Date: _____ Session: _____

Treatment: _____

Complications /
Side Effects: _____

Next Appt: _____

Date: _____ Session: _____

Treatment: _____

Complications /
Side Effects: _____

Next Appt: _____

Date: _____ Session: _____

Treatment: _____

Complications /
Side Effects: _____

Next Appt: _____

Date: _____ Session: _____

Treatment: _____

Complications /
Side Effects: _____

Next Appt: _____

Appendix D

Records

Use these pages to make sure you and your loved ones can easily locate important documents, such as health and life insurance policies, advance health care directives and powers of attorney, your will, and other records.

My Insurance Policies

Health Insurance: _____

Contact: _____

Policy #: _____

Group #: _____ ID #: _____

Rx Insurance: _____

Contact: _____

Policy #: _____

Group #: _____ ID #: _____

Vision Insurance: _____

Contact: _____

Policy #: _____

Group #: _____ ID #: _____

My Insurance Policies (Continued)

Dental Insurance: _____

Contact: _____
_____

Policy #: _____

Group #: _____ ID #: _____

Life Insurance: _____

Contact: _____
_____

Policy #: _____

Group #: _____ ID #: _____

Long-term Care: _____

Contact: _____
_____

Policy #: _____

Group #: _____ ID #: _____

Long-term Disability: _____

Contact: _____
_____

Policy #: _____

Group #: _____ ID #: _____

Other Important Documents

Type of Document	*Location*
Power of Attorney (Yes / No)	_____
Will (Yes / No)	_____
Advance Healthcare Directive—Living Will (Yes / No)	_____
Health Care Proxy (Yes / No)	_____
	_____ (Name of Proxy)
Medical Power of Attorney (Yes / No)	_____
Do Not Resuscitate Order (Yes / No)	_____
Organ / Tissue Donor (Yes / No)	_____
Instructions for Funeral / Disposal of Remains (Yes / No)	_____

About Belluck & Fox

People with mesothelioma and other asbestos-related diseases deserve justice. The attorneys at Belluck & Fox know how to obtain justice, one family at a time.

The truth is that companies knowingly exposed workers and families to deadly asbestos fibers and made them ill. Our mesothelioma lawyers stand up for those victims. We have secured more than $500 million for our clients and their families – including mesothelioma verdicts of $32 million and $19.5 million in August 2011.

Don't wait – the time for action is now. If you (or someone you dearly love) have been diagnosed with mesothelioma, put the lawyers at Belluck & Fox, LLP, to work for you. Call us at (877) 637-6843 or (212) 681-1575, or fill out the contact form online at www.belluckfox.com or www.mesotheliomahelp.net for a free consultation.

Joseph W. Belluck is a founding partner of Belluck & Fox and has extensive experience in asbestos and mesothelioma cases. He is a dedicated, compassionate attorney who has spent his entire legal career representing injured consumers and workers. Joe has a national reputation for excellence in asbestos and mesothelioma litigation. He has been recognized for both his legal work and his high ethical standards.

Jordan Fox is one of New York's most experienced product liability litigators. Jordan has represented victims of asbestos exposure for more than 25 years. He has prosecuted thousands of asbestos cases and has settled tens of millions of dollars in claims for his clients.

Belluck & Fox is nationally regarded as one of the top asbestos law firms in the United States.

Made in the USA
Middletown, DE
19 January 2019